CHINESE MEDICINE
for
BEGINNERS

CHINESE MEDICINE

for

BEGINNERS

Use the Power of the Five Elements
to Heal Body and Soul

Achim Eckert, M.D.

Prima Publishing

PRIMA PUBLISHING and colophon are registered trademarks of Prima Communications, Inc.

Note to the Reader

This book is a beginner's guide to the basic principles of Chinese medicine. It is not intended as a complete explanation of the theory and practice of Chinese medicine. While every effort has been made to illustrate each technique carefully, there can be no substitute for the supervision of a qualified practitioner of Chinese medicine. The author and publisher disclaim all responsibility for any accident or injury caused by inappropriate use of the techniques shown in this book.

Library of Congress Cataloging-in-Publication Data

Eckert, Achim
    Chinese medicine for beginners: use the power of the five elements to heal body and soul/by Achim Eckert
    ISBN 0-7615-0613-6
    1. Medicine, Chinese.   2. Hygiene, Taoist.   3. Mind and body therapies.   I. Title
R606.E23   1996
615.5'0951—dc20   96-22909
                                                                                      CIP

96 97 98 99 00 AA 10 9 8 7 6 5 4 3 2
Printed in the United States of America

How to Order:

Single copies may be ordered from Prima Publishing, P.O. Box 1260BK, Rocklin, CA 95677; telephone (916) 632-4400. Quantity discounts are also available. On your letterhead, include information concerning the intended use of the books and the number of books you wish to purchase.

Visit us online at http://www.primapublishing.com

Contents

First Steps

IN 1978, I had been studying medicine at the University of Vienna in Austria for three years. I felt that something was missing from my studies. Prior to this, an old Chinese master named *Gia-Fu Feng* had taught me *Tai Qi* (a martial art sometimes referred to as "meditation in motion") and meditation. He was the first to introduce me to the Chinese concept of *Qi*, or Life Energy. During the same time, I had participated in workshops on Reichian bodywork and Bioenergetics. My Reichian therapist talked about Orgone Energy—the Life Energy that Wilhelm Reich had discovered. And from lessons in a Yoga Ashram in Vienna, I knew about *Prana,* the Hindu concept of Life Energy. Whether doing Bioenergetic exercises, *Pranayama,* or *Tai Qi*, it all more or less amounted to the same effect: after a time of following the movements and exercises, I began to feel charged, my perception changed, and I felt happier and more alert.

So I went to India to find out more about these funny feelings of happiness in my veins and the gradual changes of perception brought on by the *Qi*-enhancing exercises and meditation techniques: colors looked brilliant, smells were overwhelming, and sounds became very clear. I was looking for an Ashram, and I found one where I stayed for a year and a half. Thereupon I went to the Maldives on a kind of Robinson Crusoe trip; I was the only white person living on the island for about two months, eating bread, fruit, rice, and coconuts, and contemplating a hundred kinds of fish.

From there, I went to Sri Lanka, where I intended to set up a gem business to finance my further stay in Asia. One evening, while watching the sunset at the beach of Mount Lavinia, a coastal village south of Colombo, I became acquainted with three German doctors who had come to Sri Lanka to study acupuncture. They, in turn, introduced me to

Professor Sir Anton Jayasuriya, who ran a government-financed acupuncture clinic; most of his patients were neither insured nor sufficiently well off to pay for treatment when sick.

For more than a year, I stayed in Sri Lanka, working and studying at the acupuncture clinic of the Colombo South Hospital. At that time, we treated between 500 and 700 patients a day. They came from all over the country, usually after the rudimentary treatments of Western medicine and the devil dance of the village had failed. In this period, I saw patients with a great variety of ailments, from asthma to elephantiasis, epilepsy to paraplegia, eczema to tinnitus, glaucoma to high blood pressure, stomatitis to gastric ulcers, and so forth. As the team consisted of an average of five doctors, I got a lot of practice with diagnosis and acupuncture needling, and acquired a routine.

I remember the first day when I came into the clinic. Professor Jayasuriya was using acupuncture to treat a patient. One of the selected points was Large Intestine 11, a point at the end of the elbow crease when the arm is flexed. With the next patient, he told me to put a needle into the same point. So I began to do acupuncture before actually knowing what I was doing. In the following weeks and months, I learned to perform acupuncture from a practical and empirical point of view— rather from instinct than from knowledge, rather from the *hara* than from the head.

Throughout this year there were not many students at the clinic. The German doctors had gone, and for some months there were two French students and a doctor from Melbourne. We rented a house on the beach together and experimented on ourselves with acupuncture and acupressure. I noticed that the needles, besides having an effect on my body and influencing my moods and emotions, gradually altered my states of consciousness; they broadened my perceptions, made my dreams more vivid and colorful, and helped to calm my mind so that I could sit at ease for hours in meditation.

In the following years, I had other teachers of Traditional Chinese Medicine. I also learned *Shiatsu* and Chinese massage. I acquired most of these skills in India and Sri Lanka and, some years later, in California. For political reasons, I never went to China. This was many years before the shootings at Tiananmen Square. I had the impression that the Communist Party of the People's Republic had removed the Taoist spiritual background from Chinese medical science. The theory of the Five Elements and the Taoist meditation techniques had been displaced by dialectic materialism, but I had left Austria in search of holistic medicine, not another materialistic view of the world.

While working at the acupuncture clinic in Colombo, I asked myself why some people immediately responded to acupuncture while others did not. I observed that people who did physical labor generally responded better to acupuncture than people who did not move much. The flow of *Qi* obviously depended on the quality of the connective tissue in the body. As the commonly used acupuncture books were not precise about the exact location of the meridians in the body, I began to think of the meridians as tiny channels, mostly running in the connective tissue between muscles and along major blood vessels and nerve-cords. The idea began to form in my mind that if it were possible to "open up" the tissue by massage, the effectiveness of acupuncture treatments could be enhanced considerably.

Later, when I learned Postural Integration in California—a method of deep-tissue structural bodywork similar to Rolfing and Heller Work—this thesis proved to be true. After giving a person ten or more sessions of deep-tissue bodywork, I would do a thorough Chinese diagnosis according to the Five Elements. This would include Chinese pulse-reading to ascertain the Fullness or Depletion of *Qi* in the various internal organs. Then I would use meridian massage to balance out Fullness and Depletion of *Qi* in the Twelve Organs and their corresponding meridians. And only if I could palpate a sufficient flow of *Qi* in the Twelve Meridians would I proceed to do acupuncture to guide the *Qi* to a place in the body, soul, and mind where it was needed—either because a symptom of a disease had remained in spite of all the bodywork and massage, or to clear up a feeling and strengthen and enhance a physical, mental, or spiritual ability.

Although many years have passed, and I have encountered a multitude of philosophies, my favored system for relating the varied phenomena of life to each other has remained the easily practicable Theory of the Five

Elements. One main reason is that it conclusively relates the material and spiritual world, the body, mind, and soul each to the others. I have not found any other theory that works as well. And since, in the Western culture, medicine, psychology, natural sciences, and religion do not have a common frame of reference, I am glad to have stumbled upon this wonderfully interconnected world-view. This integrated perspective is why I teach the Theory of the Five Elements, meridian massage, and Postural Integration, and why I wrote this book.

Introduction

IN RECENT YEARS, a notable change has occurred in the medical field. More and more people take the time to educate themselves about health: they pay attention to nutrition, they want to be physically fit, they want to feel at home in their bodies, and they try to understand what it is that makes them ill. People with a chronic illness especially prefer to be treated holistically, making use of such therapies as homeopathy, acupuncture, and the laying on of hands. Parallel to this development, the psychosomatic aspect of illness is again finding more and more resonance in the technically oriented medical field. One sign of this turning point is a tendency to treat the indivual as a whole being; body, mind, and soul are seen as an inseparable unit. This means that every physical illness denotes an underlying imbalance in the psyche or soul and must be treated accordingly.

This book was written from such an encompassing point of view—as a broad look at a world in which nature and humans are not separate, where philosophy and religion, psychology and medicine, and knowledge and wisdom go hand in hand—from a holistic understanding of people and our environment, health and disease, and body and soul.

part 1

Basic Concepts of Chinese Medicine

MANY readers may be familiar with the basic terminology of Chinese medicine. However, I would like to provide a brief introduction for those who do not have this background.

Yin and Yang

ALTHOUGH these terms are widely known, they are frequently used in an imprecise way. One of the main reasons is that the Chinese and Japanese views on Yin and Yang differ greatly. Many people nowadays might follow the Japanese practices of *Shiatsu* or macrobiotics on the one hand, and on the other hand get Chinese herbal treatments and acupuncture, causing the notions of Yin and Yang to become fuzzy at times.

The principle of Yin and Yang is an Oriental way of seeing reality that views every aspect of the world, material and spiritual, as being composed of two opposing and at the same time interdependent forces: Yin and Yang. This dualistic thinking is not unknown to us. Occidental culture, Greek science and philosophy, and Judeo-Christian religions are built on dual principles; we encounter this in the concept of matter and energy in physics, in the ideas of good and bad and heaven and hell in Christian and Islamic religions, and in the binary code of our computer world. This could be a major reason why many aspects of Chinese and Japanese culture have been received more easily in the West than those from, for example, the Dogon in Central Africa.

However, it is important to understand that the Far Eastern concept of Yin and Yang also differs from Western dualism. Yin and Yang are opposites that form a whole; they depend on each other because they only exist in relation to their opposite. The Yin-Yang symbol depicts the universal law of change. It tells us that one changes into the other at its extremes. The Yin-and-Yang symbol, each part with a dot of the opposite color in its center, represents two poles which contain at their innermost core the essence of the opposite. In other words, nothing is merely Yin or Yang, black or white, female or male, receptivity or giving, darkness or light, bad or good. This means that there are some male qualities in women and some female qualities in men—that there are always shades of gray, and that a "bad" action is never only "bad" and a "good" action may have "bad" consequences.

Yin and Yang are not absolute terms. They are always used in a relative way, describing the relationships between the various phenomena of the material and spiritual world. To give you an example: in the body, the chest is viewed as Yin in comparison with the back, but in comparison with the pelvis the chest is Yang. Or another example: in comparison with daytime, the night is viewed as Yin, but in comparison with a black hole, our night on earth is Yang because it still contains some light.

In Western culture, there is a tendency to take things that are relatives as absolutes. We have been educated to see things as either good or bad. But Yin and Yang cannot be categorized as either good or bad. The Yin-Yang symbol represents the way things change; it is a description, not a judgment. It tells us how opposites depend on each other, how they embrace each other, and how they finally become each other.

The following list of Yin and Yang attributes expresses the Chinese view and might differ considerably from the Japanese use of the terms. When using the list of Yin and Yang attributes, it is also important to remember the relative nature of the described opposites.

GENERAL ATTRIBUTES

Yin	Yang
matter	energy
proton	electron
centripetal force	centrifugal force
contraction	expansion
downward direction	upward direction
earth	heaven
horizontal	vertical

continues

General Attributes

Yin	Yang
darkness	light
night	day
cold	heat
moon	sun
silver	gold
winter	summer
end	beginning
old	young
negative	positive
passive	active
female	male
soft	hard
in-flow	out-flow
rest	movement
slow	fast
interior	exterior
receptivity	giving
wet	dry
gravity	growth
roots, trunk	branches, leaves
fruit	sprout, shoot
alkaline	acid

Body and Mind

Yin	Yang
front	back
left side	right side
lower body	upper body
trunk	limbs
legs	arms
pelvis	head
solid organs (*Zang*)	hollow organs (*Fu*)
organs	meridians
Yong Qi	*Wei Qi*
blood	energy

continues

BODY AND MIND

Yin	Yang
sensory system	motor system
flexion	extension
rest and regeneration	movement and action
digestion and reproduction	fight or flight
parasympathetic nervous system	sympathetic nervous system
acetylcholine	adrenaline
heart rythm	respiratory rythm
inhalation	exhalation
instinct	intelligence
feeling	will
intuition	intellect
introversion	extroversion
quiet, calm	talkative, agitated
grounded	experimental
conservative	progressive
contemplative	excitable, reactive
depressed	elated

PATHOLOGY

Yin	Yang
chronic	acute
internal diseases	skin diseases and disorders of the sensory organs
degenerative diseases	infections
pale face	red face
hypersalivation	dry mouth
no thirst	thirsty
likes warm drink	prefers cold drink
cool body	hot body
edema	inflammation and fever
slow and weak reaction	fast and strong reaction to bacteria and viruses
paralysis	convulsions
numbness	spasms
flacidity	cramps
abundant menstruation	scanty menstruation

continues

PATHOLOGY

Yin	Yang
long menstrual cycle	short menstrual cycle
prefers quiet	likes to move
tiny voice	loud voice
moist skin	dry skin
puffy skin	scaly skin
diarrhea	constipation

PAIN

Yin	Yang
chronic	acute
old	recent
permanent	intermittent
deep	superficial
diffuse, extended	localized
dull, heavy	sharp, pulsating, itching, shooting
worse at nighttime	*worse in the* daytime
worsened by rest	*worsened by* motion
worse in cold	*worse in* heat
better in daytime	*better at* nighttime
made better by motion	made *better by* rest
better in heat	*better in* cold
soft touch	firm pressure

MASSAGE

Treating a Yin Condition	Treating a Yang Condition
gentle	firm
quick strokes	slow strokes
superficial	deep
upward	downward
clockwise	counterclockwise
short duration (up to half an hour)	long duration (an hour or more)
with the nails and fingertips	with the thumbs, palms, elbows, and feet

The Chinese View
of the Organs

THE Chinese view of the internal organs and body tissues differs from the Western concept. This is because Chinese culture does not separate body and soul. According to Chinese medicine, each organ has, in addition to its physical function, an emotional, mental, and spiritual function. Soul and mind are not just based in the brain, but are in every cell in the body and in the entire energy field of the organism. The inner organs are interpreted more as a body-mind-spirit unit than as an anatomical form with physiological functions. Thus, each organ makes a contribution to the whole personality, and its interactions with other organs are of utmost importance to the mental and emotional levels.

Because the organs are not looked upon from a merely physiological standpoint, but from an elemental point of view that considers body, mind, and spirit as the expression of five elemental forces and their constant interplay, the anatomical definitions of the internal organs also differ from those of Western medicine. For example: the stomach, the duodenum, and the first six inches of the small intestine, in Western terms, are jointly called the Stomach in Chinese medicine. This is because the Chinese consider the digestive process and the absorption of nutrients from the digestive tract into the bloodstream as the main task of the Stomach. To make a clear distinction between the Chinese and Western organ concepts, the organs, according to Chinese under-standing, are spelled with capital initial letters in this book. Another example: the Chinese Spleen consists of not only the spleen, but also the pancreas and all the lymphatic tissue and organs in the body. The reason is that the physical duty of the Spleen is to maintain the sub-stance of the body. For this purpose, the pancreas, which produces most of the digestive juices, and all of the organs and cells that constitute the immune system—such as tonsils, lymph glands, and spleen—are com-bined in one organ: the Spleen.

ZANG AND FU ORGANS

Chinese medicine differentiates between six Yin and six Yang organs. The Yin organs are called *Zang*: the character *zang* means "firm" or "solid." The six *Zang* have a firmer consistency than the six *Fu*. They are also called storage organs because, in addition to their physiological functions, they take up different forms of *Qi* (life energy) and store, produce, or transform them. The six *Zang* organs are the Heart, the Pericardium, the Liver, the Kidney, the Lung, and the Spleen.

The six Yang organs are called *Fu*: the sign *fu* means "hollow." The hol-low organs are the Stomach, Small Intestine, Large Intestine, Gall Blad-der, Urinary Bladder, and Triple Warmer. The main tasks of the *Fu* are the reception and digestion of food, the absorption of nutrients, and the excretion of waste products. The duties of the Triple Warmer are the reg-ulation of the temperature in the body and the coordination of the func-tions of the chest, stomach, and pelvis: the coordination of breathing, circulation, digestion, elimination, and sexuality.

Each *Zang* organ is paired with a *Fu* organ of the same element. Their physiological, emotional, intellectual, and spiritual functions are closely related; each *Zang* organ embodies the Yin power, each *Fu* the Yang force of the corresponding element.

Meridians

THE meridians are the channels that *Qi*, the life force or vital energy, flows through, and the acupressure or acupuncture points are the places where you can tap into that energy flow.

Traditional Chinese medicine views the meridians as a network connecting the interior with the exterior: the internal organs with the surface of the body, tissue with spirit, Yin with Yang, earth with sky. It is a system of energy channels running mainly along the long axis of the body, with the exception of the *Luo* vessels and the *Dai Mai,* an extraordinary channel that circles the waist like a belt. For this reason, the meridian system was compared by Western doctors to the meridian system of the earth: The organ meridians correspond with the earth's longitudinal meridians, the *Luo* vessels with the latitudinal meridians, and the *Dai Mai* with the equator.

In the *Huang Di Nei Jing,* the Yellow Emperor's Classic of Internal Medicine which dates back to approximately the third century before Christ, the pathway of the meridians and the effects of the acupuncture points were already precisely and extensively described. In this text, the meridians are compared to the big rivers and streams of China which irrigate and fertilize the land. The Chinese character for meridian is *jing,* meaning "river, path, track, or trail," and also "blood vessel."

The meridian system consists mainly of the Twelve Organ Meridians, also called the Twelve Regular Channels. Each of the Twelve Organ Meridians pertains to and connects with a particular *Zang* or *Fu* organ;

the organ meridian is the main energy channel that connects the particular organ with other organs and the surface of the body.

The Twelve Organ Meridians form pairs. Each Yin meridian is assigned to a Yang meridian of the same element. These pairs are also called Coupled Meridians, because their *Qi* flow is kept in balance by two sluice gates. These floodgates are the *Luo* vessels which form, together with the organ meridians, the network of channels that I mentioned above. Connecting the Coupled Meridians, their task is to ensure that the energy flow of Coupled Meridians is level, thus reducing the risk of an excess or deficiency of *Qi* in the particular meridian and its pertaining organ. The Chinese character *luo* means "to connect," "to link," "to tie together and network."

The function of the meridians and the *Luo* vessels is to provide a circulation of *Qi* throughout the body, thus nourishing the tissues and linking up the whole body so as to keep the internal organs, four limbs, muscles, tendons, and bones intact and to make the body an organic integrity.

Qi, the Life Force

QI is the Chinese name for vital energy or Life Force. Its Japanese term is *Ki*, and in Yoga it is called *Prana*. Most ancient cultures have the concept of an essential Life Force that circulates in the air, plants, animals, and the human body. It is the life behind the atom—the energy found in all forms of matter, and it is concentrated in living organisms.

Although Paracelsus and Mesmer, healers of the 16th and 18th centuries in Europe, still referred to the notion of a Life Force, this term lost importance over the course of Western medical history.

Wilhelm Reich, an Austrian doctor who later emigrated to the U.S., was the first in this century to rediscover the vital energy or Life Force in scientific experiments. He called it "Orgone energy"—and had big problems with the FDA for manufacturing and selling Orgone accumulators, leading to his imprisonment and the public burning of his books in the U.S. in the fifties. During that time, the Russians also experimented with the Life Force, calling it "bioplasma." This led to the development of Kirlian photography, with which it is possible to make the energy field of living organisms visible.

Three to four thousand years ago, Indian and Chinese cultures developed systems of healing and meditation to enhance vital energy in people in order to prevent disease and to heal the sick. The Chinese discerned various kinds of Life Force or *Qi*.

The most important terms for us to understand, in relation to *Qi*, are *Shi* and *Xu*. *Shi* means Fullness or Excess of energy, leading mostly to

Yang or Hot symptoms such as inflammation, pain, and fever. *Xu* means Depletion or Deficiency of energy, resulting mostly in Yin or Cold symptoms such as chills, edema, numbness, and chronic pain. The meridian exercises that are described later in this book are used to balance out an excess or a deficiency of *Qi* in the various meridians and their corresponding organs, thus enhancing health and well-being.

The Chinese differentiated between acquired and congenital *Qi*. The congenital *Qi* that one inherits from one's parents and ancestors is also called Ancestral Energy. The guardians of the Ancestral Energy are the kidneys.

The Ancestral Energy is needed to form the *Qi* that one receives from food and air. In the Middle Warmer, Essential Energy or *Zong Qi*, is "cooked" from food and air *Qi*; the Middle Warmer is the stove, and the Ancestral Energy is the fuel. The *Zong Qi* moves up to the chest, nourishes the Heart and Lung to promote their functions, and divides into *Yong Qi* and *Wei Qi*. *Yong Qi* is nutrient *Qi*; its function is to nourish the body and maintain its substance. *Wei Qi* is defensive energy that defends the organism against exogenous pathogenic factors.

The Five Elements

IN THE TAOIST teachings of the Five Elements, also referred to as "natural powers," the connections of the elements, the body, and the spirit are described in detail. These elements and the laws by which they operate can be observed at work in all of natural phenomena, including the human being.

In Western culture, the laws of nature concerning the physical world are formulated. They are limited to things that can be measured physically, and they cannot be used in the realms of emotions and thought, fantasy and intuition. As a result, our culture is often described as one-sided. As rich, precise, and varied as our knowledge of the material world may be, our knowledge of the psyche and the mental world is limited, confused, and speculative. Most of the time we are not even aware of how limited our thoughts are. Studying the *I-Ching* (The Book of Changes) or the spiritual world of the Tibetan Lamas, Japanese Zen masters, or Native American shamans can show us that dimensions exist beyond the psychological and religious knowledge of Western culture.

In ancient China, the laws of nature were formulated so that the observed phenomena of both the material world and the spiritual world could be explained, and a relationship between them could be established. The separation into a material and nonmaterial world did not arise, at least not in our sense. At that time, the world was seen as an interplay of spirits and demons, of powers and forces of nature.

As in all cultures that are not "protected" by technology, these ancient people both respected and feared the forces of nature: the drought-bringing heat of the summer, the typhoons, the tidal waves, the rage of the gods in the thunder. It was common to call on the guardian spirits and to placate the demons. Earth, fire, heaven, and water were gods. One had to be aware of their signals if one wanted to survive.

These people began to observe and collect experiences, which they passed on from generation to generation. They observed the cycles of life, the courses of the stars, and the changes of weather; they observed these natural phenomena in connection with human beings, with their feelings and ways of thinking, with their dreams and their illnesses.

Out of these observations crystallized the teachings of the *Tao*. The *Tao* is also called "the unnameable"—that from which everything is born, yet that which has no direction, no will, no goal: that which is. The polarities are born out of the *Tao*: Yin and Yang, earth and heaven, matter and energy. The Five Elements are born from Yin and Yang. In their image they bring forth, create, maintain, and break down the world.

It is important to understand that our term "element" does not have the same meaning as the Chinese term. The Chinese see an element, not as a material substance, but rather as a power—a specific quality of the universe. As the translation shows, this term is not limited to the power of nature, but refers in general to its laws and principles. The elements are seen as transition phases of the varied manifestations of *Qi*—as energetic states that return again and again. The Chinese idea of transition phases and energetic states corresponds to modern discoveries in physics in an amazing way, especially to the idea of energy fields, quantum mechanics, and the Heisenberg Uncertainty Principle. Scientists such as Niels Bohr and Fritjof Capra have recognized the similarity between quantum physics and the Taoist world-view (see *The Tao of Physics,* by Fritjof Capra).

According to Chinese views, the Five Elements are evident in all manifestations in the cosmos: in the directions, the seasons, the climate, the stars, the plants and animals, the mineral and rock layers, and human beings. The senses, organs, and tissues of living beings are assigned to elements, as are emotions and mental abilities. The elements are powers that keep each other balanced; they create each other; they change into and block one another. If the energetic relationships of the elements are not balanced, this expresses itself in a human being as discomfort and illness, and in a society as weakness, injustice, and war. If the elements in a person—as well as in a society or a state—are balanced and strong, one finds harmony and health, beauty and grace.

In reading about the Five Elements, it may be helpful to refer to the chart "Classification by the Five Elements" at the back of this book.

part 2

WOOD

The Element Wood

THE STRENGTH of Wood manifests itself in the morning and in the east, in birth and in every new undertaking, in the freshness of the wind and in spring. In the Chinese tradition, the elements form a cycle; this will be explained extensively in Part VII. Wood is the first element of the cycle. It is called the "young Yang." In the body, Wood manifests itself in the Liver and Gall Bladder, in the muscles and tendons, in the eyes and in their tears. The Liver and Gall Bladder produce the emotions that are ascribed to Wood: irritability, anger, fury, and rage. In the spirit, Wood brings forth the desire for movement and growth; it brings forth the creative process—planning and decision-making—and it gives us the desire to untertake a new project, to set sail for new horizons and new discoveries. The color associated with Wood is green.

The key to understanding this element is seen in the tree. The tree is rooted in the earth, often as deeply as its branches reach into the sky. Through its roots, the tree takes in water and minerals for its nourishment. It grows high into the sky, branches reaching out in all directions. The tree has always symbolized growth in every direction: above and below, to the east and to the west, to the north and to the south. It has long been a symbol of expansive energy. In fall and in winter, it draws back into itself and gathers strength for a new spring and summer, for a new growth ring.

Many ancient cultures worshipped the tree. Many considered the tree to be inhabited by spirits, for example in China or in the Celtic culture. The Germans worshipped the oak. And the Essenes, a religious sect in ancient Palestine, portrayed the human being in the center of the tree of life: connected to energy lines as if in a magnetic field, the human stood in relation to the powers of heaven and earth. The figure was drawn in a meditative pose, the upper half of its body being the branches extending over the earth, and the lower half being the roots growing into the earth. The positions of the physical organs were also portrayed. The digestive, eliminative, and reproductive organs in the lower half of the body represented the earthly component. The lungs, heart, and brain in the upper half of the body connected the person with the powers of the heavens. But the liver and gall bladder—the Wood organs—were portrayed at the center of the body, connecting what is above with what is below. Thus it appears that cultures other than the Chinese saw the connection between the liver and the tree.

The liver is the Yin organ of the element Wood. Thus, it embodies the Yin energy of Wood: the ability to plan and see life on a material level as well as on an intellectual and spiritual level. The liver embodies the power of imagination, the creative energy in us that results in growth. It is the inventor, the discoverer. It sees the meaning of life. It develops the vision, the plan. Every new idea that we take hold of, every new concept, broadens our horizons. We take risks and go into the unknown. We grow.

When the element Wood is healthy and balanced in someone, this person is able to see that nature embodies an immense plan in which everything has its place and its role—everything that happens, even the seemingly small and meaningless things, contributes to the pattern of events.

The cosmic plan goes beyond our power of imagination to such an extent that often we can perceive the connection and inner meaning of a chain of events only after a long time has passed. As long as we trust the cosmic plan, we keep a deep connection to the world. We grow with our environment, not against it.

The Yang organ of Wood is the gall bladder. It embodies the Yang energy of this element: our ability to make decisions and to assert our needs in the outer world. One can compare the liver to an architect who designs a house, while the gall bladder is the builder who makes the decisions and arrangements that are necessary for the house to become a reality. The functions of both organs are closely connected to each other. Without an all-encompassing concept, the decisions in day-to-day life are incoherent, making little sense. At the same time, the best plans and projects are worthless if they cannot be carried out.

If planning and organization become a dry, bureaucratic routine, they will not lead to growth, but will often bring more harm than good. In the language of the Five Elements, inflexible and rigid planning is labeled "dry Wood," because it cracks and breaks under minimal pressure. Wood must be supple and full of sap so that real growth is possible.

In order to carry out a plan, we must take steps to realize it. We must "come out of ourselves" and fetch what we need to live. Therefore, it is understandable that the muscles and tendons are the bodily tissues assigned to Wood. If there is an obstacle to our growth—if we cannot find the space for expression—we feel frustrated and become angry. Anger and aggression are signs that our life energy is blocked, either from without or from within. In the theory of the Five Elements, anger and aggression are seen in a positive light: as emotions that help us to overcome impediments to our growth. Anger and aggression are the expression of a healthy Wood element, whereas irritability, hatred, rage, and fury are perceived as signs of an imbalance in Wood.

Rage and fury can be seen as undefined forms of aggression, with few possibilities for expression through language, gestures, or actions. Many people who feel constant rage lack the ability to recognize conflicts within themselves and express them to others. These people often did not learn in childhood to express their needs so as to receive what they wanted; their rage or fury built up over the years. Because they are often not capable of seeing their problems clearly, one also speaks of "blind rage." Rage is anger that has lost its purpose and gone out of control. Fury and rage typically lead to destructive behavior.

If rage is kept inside and cannot be cleared out, it seethes under a cold, numb, often polite surface. When it breaks out, it can become dangerous, as we all know. So it happens, again and again, that well-behaved, seemingly well-adjusted people commit murder or suicide in a fit of desperation.

Anger stands in contrast to rage. Anger is an energy that moves in the upper half of the body. It has more direction and focus than rage; it can be more easily expressed. As mentioned above, anger helps us to clear obstacles out of our way so that we can carry through with our plans. In situations where the reason for being angry seems justified, one speaks of a "holy wrath." A well-known example of this is the scene in the Old Testament in which Moses comes down with the Ten Commandments from Mount Sinai and finds the Jews dancing around the golden calf, praying to an idol. As we know, he was overcome by a holy wrath that had important consequences for the further development of Judaism.

Annoyance and irritability are also ascribed to the Wood element. They are emotional energies that also move in the upper half of the body but, in contrast to anger, they are often symptoms of an emotional process in the unconscious; the energy has not yet been focused. In the language of the Five Elements, this is termed as "Wood which has not yet been gathered."

Anger, rage, and fury are seen in Chinese medicine as expressions of the Wood Yang. A choleric temperament, chronic irritability, and unreasonable temper tantrums indicate a *Shi* state of the gall bladder (a gall bladder in the state of Fullness of *Qi*), which can also manifest itself as severe migraines in the temples or at the crown of the head. A longstanding *Shi* state of the gall bladder—a rage that cannot be clearly expressed and cleared out—often leads to high blood pressure or gall stones.

A lack of Yang energy in Wood leads to suppressed rage, sarcasm, cynicism, bitterness, and, in general, an inability to get angry. It expresses itself in apathy, sluggishness, resignation, and depression. In these cases, there is too much Yin energy in Wood, either through an overactivity of Yin in the liver or through a lack of Yang in the gall bladder.

The deep bitterness of people who have been gravely disappointed in life is the result of long years of frustration, usually stemming from being confronted constantly with obstacles to self-realization. It shows a long-existing imbalance in Wood. Irony, sarcasm, and cynicism are found in people who, often in their early childhood, lost the ability to easily approach and interact with other people. They are often the products of a strict intellectual or puritanical upbringing in which the expression of emotions and physical contact was taboo.

Apathy, resignation, and depression show that a person has given up making plans and manifesting goals. This outlook arises from continued failure; a person who is unable to act independently or to carry through with something eventually gives up. This often leads to alcoholism and addiction to drugs that are destructive to the liver, as medication often is. In the Chinese tradition, the liver is seen as the "House of Hun" or the "House of the Soul"—and the soul has become apathetic. Alcohol contributes to the maintenance of this condition, in which there is no room for new hopes that would question the aquired dismal view of the world.

Depression and resignation often have their roots in a disorder in Wood. The vision is missing, the plan is lacking (a lack of Qi in the liver). Or a person might have many wishes and ideas, but just cannot put them into reality (a lack of Qi in the gall bladder). As the Qi flows in the body from the Liver to the Lung meridian, a lack of Qi in the liver eventually leads to a depletion of Qi in the lungs, causing shallow breathing, a sunken chest, and collapsed shoulders.

If, over the years, emotions such as hatred or rage cannot be expressed, cleared, and turned into a positive striving toward individual goals, the aggresion often directs itself against one's own body. This can lead to illnesses such as gout, arthritis, rheumatism, and chronic polyarthritis—diseases in which the main symptoms are joint and muscle pains and an increasing restriction of movement.

Autoimmune diseases are also becoming more widespread and varied. In these illnesses, the body's cells produce antibodies that attack its own tissue. These are also appropriately called auto-aggressive diseases. The illnesses develop over years and decades; they are chronic and can be treated symptomatically by Western medical practices and eventually brought to a standstill, but they do not go away through medication. These diseases are found most often in women. In patriarchal cultures, women have less room than men to move and express themselves, especially when it comes to carrying through with an idea or venting anger.

To summarize, it is important for us to understand that, in the teachings of the Five Elements, anger and aggression are not put on the same level as destructive behavior, but rather understood as a basic impulse—as the energy of Wood. The word "aggression" comes from the Latin verb *aggredi,* which means "to approach or tackle a thing or a person." If this normal expression of approaching someone or tackling something is hindered or restricted, it leads to a build-up of emotion; in the body it leads to stiff muscles. This muscle tension is found, above all, in the neck, back, shoulders, and arms. Accumulated aggression is one of the major causes of headaches, neck pain, and back pain.

The growth of Wood occurs in all directions. If it has the necessary space and nourishment, then it grows balanced and symmetrical. Coordination and symmetry are essential characteristics of this element in nature, as well as in the lives of human beings. Most diseases in which symptoms occur only in one half of the body, or those distinguished by a lack of coordination of the muscles, glands, and organs, can be traced to a disturbance in the element Wood. Frequently, one can see an imbalance in Wood or can recognize it through an asymmetry in the face, or in the build of the body, or in a strong difference between the visual strength of the two eyes.

Because Wood governs the cycles of growth, when it is not balanced it causes disturbances such as growth disorders in childhood and puberty, irregular or painful menstruation, premature birth, or cancer. Other physical consequences of an imbalance in Wood are diseases of the eyes and problems with vision. These include near-sightedness and astigmatism (far-sightedness related to the aging process is more of a physiological development resulting from the tiring of the Wood element in later years). Other characteristic illnesses are high blood pressure and headaches behind the eyes, in the temples, and at the crown of the head.

In the psychiatric and neurological area, an imbalance in Wood is exhibited in various mental disorders, especially in schizophrenia and some forms of epilepsy. Schizophrenia is an expression of a split personality; an essential role of Wood is to bring mental, spiritual, and physical components into equilibrium by coordinating the right and left hemispheres of the brain. To a lesser degree, many people in our culture suffer from impaired coordination of the left and right hemispheres of the brain; this is reflected in the growing number of people who need psychotherapy and heavy medication to stay balanced. This results, in part, from an educational system that primarily trains the left side of the brain. As a consequence, in recent decades people are having more and more difficulty bringing thought, logic, and rationality into harmony with intuition, fantasy, creativity, and feelings.

With epilepsy, the process is complex. Several elements contribute to the evolution of this disease. In most cases, epilepsy occurs because the relationship between Fire and Water is disturbed. If the Water element in a person has weakened, Water cannot put out the Fire (see Part VII, on The Four Cycles) and, in certain stressful situations, the Fire blazes too high. This results in an epileptic fit, which is nothing but a short circuit in the brain.

The connection between epilepsy and the Wood element lies in the similarity between a major temper tantrum and an epileptic fit, as well as in a deeper spiritual process that takes place during a fit and can perhaps only be completely understood by a shaman. I would like to point out that many seers and prophets, such as Moses, were epileptics or showed similar symptoms while in trance. Many ancient cultures view epilepsy as a holy illness that allows the soul to enter into a dimension similar to that of the hereafter.

As emphasized by the list of diseases and disorders connected with Wood, this element is of great importance not only in diagnosis and therapy, but also to better understand many diseases caused by civilization, such as migraines, menstrual disorders, visual problems, and high blood pressure. Most important, the increasingly common auto-aggressive diseases (in which the element Earth plays an important role along with Wood), are not completely understood by Western medical practitioners. They probably cannot be grasped in their entirety by a materially oriented culture, because the causes lie mostly on mental and spiritual levels. Often these causes weaken an organ so much that infections or other illnesses can develop.

With disorders in Wood, the treatment can be difficult because Wood is the element of the hypochondriac. This makes sense if one considers that confusion and disorder reign when plans and decisions are lacking. In such cases, symptoms come and go, or they seem to wander naturally from one part of the body to another. A weak constitution and symptoms that always appear in spring also indicate a Wood-related illness, as spring is the time when Wood releases its strength.

When Wood is balanced, springtime brings new interests and goals along with ambition and vitality. In contrast, when Wood is sick, spring will be a time of frustration, bringing tiredness and depression. Statistics show that the suicide rate rises in the spring. With a traditional treatment according to the teachings of the Five Elements, it is possible to restore balance so that new growth can be promoted. Then the vital energy that spring brings to Wood can carry through into the warmth of summer, the ripening period of late summer, the harvest time of fall, and the restful period of winter, when seeds can begin to germinate in preparation for a new cycle of growth.

Just as it is possible to see the workings of the Five Elements on a person's physical, mental, and spiritual levels, one can also see their influence in interpersonal relations in different cultural and social structures. Cultural, national, and social systems create structures analogous to the human organism. Several ancient civilizations see our earth as an enormous organism, with humankind as the central nervous system. This analogy makes it clear how easily the breakdown of a part of this gigantic central nervous system jeopardizes the well-being of the total organism.

In Europe, North America, and Japan, the worst consequences of an imbalance in Wood can be observed. In these highly industrialized countries, a schism exists in the relationship with this Element. In the language of the Elements, the division can be described as a very strong, self-conscious Wood-Yang that is pitted against a weak, undernourished, confused Wood-Yin.

On the one hand, these countries have been expanding magnificently for a long time. They have made technological advances, built strong military forces, and spread their religions. They have imposed their wills and their world-views onto many other peoples. Many inventions and discoveries have arisen out of these cultures. On the other hand, it is striking to witness the meaninglessness and growing insecurity that plague many people in the large, developed cities of these "advanced" regions. And there is a deep-seated confusion and lack of direction in connection with the global discussion of ecology, the dying out of the forests, and the debate about nuclear weapons.

There is a lot of discussion and a lot of information, but no vision. These discussions deliver many messages, but without much mature contemplation. The ability to have visions and to recognize how things are connected is no longer respected, and because of this, it is not developed. Visionaries are handled with mistrust; Socrates and Christ were poisoned and crucified. Others were slandered, not understood, put in prison, silenced, or executed. There are numerous examples: witches and magicians in the Middle Ages, Paracelsus, Franz Anton Mesmer, Georg Büchner, Friedrich Nietzsche, Sigmund Freud, Wilhelm Reich, Gandhi, and Martin Luther King Jr., to name a few. In other cultures, a certain amount of unusual behavior from seers and prophets was endured or even encouraged. They were given the right to criticize and inform the ruling party; this was permitted of court fools in the Middle Ages. On the contrary, in our culture, wise men and fools are ridiculed.

Vision is the power of Wood. Usually, before a new vision can take shape, confusion, dissolution, and chaos rule. In other cultures, therefore, the elders both tolerated the temperament of the fools and respected their wisdom. A further crossroads in our relationship with Wood manifests itself in our attitude toward aggression. On the one hand, aggression is described in Christian teachings as being bad and wicked. In interpersonal relationships, a loud word or a strong gesture is frequently judged negatively. The natural expression of playful aggression was often restricted and suppressed in childhood.

On the other hand, Western culture is one of the most aggressive cultures that has ever existed. It has "made the world its subject," as the Bible puts it. The extent of the destruction that has been inflicted by this culture does not need to be described here. The curbing and suppression of aggression in interpersonal relationships has led to an enormous build-up of rage that discharges itself again and again on a cultural and national level. So we find ourselves in a paradoxical situation, in which the leaders of the industrialized world speak about peace and safety, and instead give birth to destruction. They bring advancement and progress to other cultures, thus destroying them. Most scientific theories of aggression tend not to account for the effect of aggression on a national and cultural level.

Aggression is our "blind spot"; it is judged by orthodox psychology as pathological and destructive, as something that should be treated and transformed.

Another current opinion in Western culture is that anger and aggression should be sublimated and transformed into love and peace. This would be ideal, but it only works if the anger has been properly expressed and has turned naturally to joy and love. We can watch this phenomenon with small children who, after a brisk and rough fight, become easily reconciled with each other. If the anger is supressed and not expressed, and people try to be kind and polite under all circumstances, real feelings are replaced by unnatural behavior patterns. This often results in a false spirituality, in which creativity and spontaneity are subtly cut off and slowly vanish from the personality.

A further cause of the negativity projected onto aggression lies in its close association with sexuality. As observed in the investigations of anthropologists and researchers such as Margaret Mead and Wilhelm Reich, inhibited and suppressed aggression goes hand in hand with inhibited and suppressed sexuality. Stated in positive terms, healthy aggressive behavior is a condition of healthy sexual behavior, and healthy sexual behavior is related to healthy aggressive behavior.

This connection is also portrayed in the paintings of the Chinese: Wood naturally expands, flowing gently, continuously, and unimpeded. If you love someone physically, spiritually, or intellectually, you extend yourself into that person's space. When you hug another person, the space you are in expands. This simple phenomenon of gentle expansion and connecting with another—creating a larger space than the separate self—is love, which belongs to the element Wood.

The problems that Western culture has with Wood show themselves here also. On the one hand, love is highly prized and mystified, yet on the other hand, it is restricted and detached from the physical. Conditions are placed on the avenues of its expression and it is clothed in strict rituals. The flower children of the sixties were pursued and discriminated against by the police. "Make love not war!" stood for an anticultural, immoral provocation.

Interestingly, the term "love" rarely shows up in old Chinese texts. In the *I-Ching*—The Book of Changes—there is no hexagram that represents our idea of love. There is Peace, The Receptive, The Creative, The Aroused, The Gentle, The Serene, and The Obliging, but our concept of love does not appear. Only in the newer commentaries on the *I-Ching* does one find this term.

In an ancient Chinese text called the *Da Dsuan,* The Large Discourse, it is written:

> In that the person becomes like the heavens and the earth, he does not come to be opposed to them. His wisdom embraces all things and his mind orders the whole world. Because of this, he does not make any mistakes. He has an effect on everything, but he does not let himself be carried away by anything. He is joyful of the heavens and knows fate. Thus, he is free of worries. He is satisfied with his situation and sincere in his goodness. Therefore, he is capable of expressing love.

Mental and Physical Exercises to Stimulate the Growth of Wood

WHILE reading this section, you have probably already noticed some information that is relevant to your own life. Perhaps you have also asked yourself how this knowledge can influence your health, your feelings, or your world-view.

It makes a big difference whether you read about the art of running and its positive effects and then find the time and energy to run, or if you allow the theory to be enough. In order to go beyond an intellectual understanding of the elements, I have put together some exercises to give you direct experience with each element. With these, you can touch, hear, smell, taste, and see things that the printed word cannot convey. These experiences take place in your body and become anchored in your senses and movements; they become integrated into your self.

CLARIFYING QUESTIONS

The questions in this chapter have to do with your Wood element. You will find out in which areas you depart from the description of "healthy Wood."

Give yourself at least half an hour without interruptions to calmly and thoughtfully answer all of the following questions. Make yourself comfortable. Read a question, then close your eyes and let the question sink into you. Our waking consciousness is often ready to give quick answers that are only partially true. Pay attention to the first answer that comes into your head and to paradoxical answers that do not seem to fit into the picture.

Life is a state of maintaining relative balance between various constantly changing imbalances. Small deviations from the norm are typical of a lively life. In all areas of our existence, we sway back and forth between two poles. If we remain stuck on the Yin or Yang pole for any length of time and we do not express the other pole, our growth and maturation will be restricted and our physical and mental health will be harmed. Examples of opposite poles are: waking vs. sleeping, relaxed vs. active or tense, anger vs. gentleness.

Use the following questions to get to know the condition of your Wood element and to discover any imbalances you may have. For example, there is something wrong with your Wood element if you are always irritable and you explode at the slightest provocation, but there is also something wrong if you are unable to get angry at all in a situation in which people seriously mistreat you. Some other examples: there is something wrong with your Wood if you have major vision problems; if you either cannot stand sour tastes or you have a deep craving for sour food; or if you easily get irritable and hysterical in windy weather.

These questions cannot simply be answered by "yes" or "no," and nobody is there to tell you how many points you have scored in the Wood element. Use these questions to develop a sense of whether your Wood element is more or less balanced. If you get the impression that your Wood element is either too strong or too weak, do the subsequent exercises that can help you to win back your balance. If you want to experience a change, do the mental and emotional exercises such as "Vision of the Future" and "Unexpressed Anger" a few times within a month, and do the exercises to stimulate the flow of *Qi* in the Liver and Gall Bladder Meridians on a daily basis for three weeks.

- How do I feel in the morning?
- How do I feel in spring?

Mental and Physical Exercises to Stimulate the Growth of Wood

- How do I feel on windy days?
- Do I have a special craving for or a strong aversion to sour food or drink?
- Are my liver and gall bladder healthy, or have I had jaundice, gall stones, or a bilious attack?
- Do I have strong or weak muscles?
- Do I enjoy movement?
- Am I active in sports?
- Do I have a tendency toward inflamed tendons or pulled muscles?
- Am I sometimes paralyzed in situations, but do not let anything show and become angry after the fact?
- How do I express anger and frustration?
- How often do I swallow anger instead of exploding?
- Am I often ironic or cynical?
- Is there something in my personal history that gives me bitter feelings?
- Do I frequently feel a thirst for revenge?
- Do I hate somebody?
- Am I often irritable or moody?
- Can I attain my goals and carry through with my intentions most of the time?
- Do I have a picture of how I would like to live, and does my reality correspond to that picture?
- How good is my eyesight?
- How do I approach new situations?

WOOD EXERCISES

VISION OF THE FUTURE   Spend an evening alone. Take a bath and put on light, comfortable clothes. Seek a quiet place where you can relax undisturbed.

Lie on your back, close your eyes, and breathe deeply and regularly for about a minute, like a sleeping child. Then imagine that you are journeying into the picture of your life that you carry within you. Paint the details of how you would like to live. Dream yourself into a world where there are no restrictions or limitations. If a good fairy could help you to realize your wishes, what occupation would you like to have? With which partner would you live? How much time would you have for yourself and your personal interests? How would your relationships with other people be?

Do not let yourself be disturbed at this time by negative or critical thoughts. Ignore the doubter, the one who is resigned and cynical. Every thought can become reality, but you have to give it time to take root and develop.

The best time for a future vision is in February or March, but you can do this exercise at other times, especially before making important decisions. A vision gains strength when you write it down in a journal and when you visualize it often in vivid detail.

UNEXPRESSED ANGER If you have difficulty venting your anger in the presence of other people, try the following exercise:

Withdraw to a room or look for a place in the open air where you will not be disturbed. Imagine a concrete situation in which you did not dare to let your anger run free. See the person with whom you were in conflict symbolically in a pillow. Spontaneously express your opinion as if the person were standing directly in front of you. Allow yourself to become powerful, to raise your voice, shout, rant, and become physical. Exaggerate a bit and let yourself go in the situation.

EVERYDAY IRRITATION Practice expressing aggressive behavior for a few days. Invite situations that arouse your anger and seek meetings with people who you know will drive you up a wall. Express your anger energetically. Observe yourself when you are angry. Observe the reactions of others. Is it how you thought it would be?

I know this is a tough one. The purpose of the exercise is to de-automatize the way you deal with difficulties and hindrances. If you have a difficult time getting angry at all, this exercise should prove to be particularly helpful: you "exercise" an assertive response to have it on hand when you really need it. Because in the actual situation where there is a major difficulty, there are always multiple reasons to not speak up.

If you are a hothead, this exercise is helpful in order to become conscious of your anger patterns. If you deliberately set up a situation in which to become angry, you are beginning to master your aggression

Mental and Physical Exercises to Stimulate the Growth of Wood

and your anger pattern will change because awareness transforms the automatic emotional response.

MOVEMENT   Physical movement that causes perspiration strengthens the element Wood. Along with heavy physical work, most sports fulfill this purpose. Martial arts (for example Judo, Karate, and Aikido) especially strengthen a weak Wood element and combat excess body weight.

EXERCISES FOR THE GALL BLADDER AND LIVER MERIDIANS

You know how it is with exercises. We would rather think about them than do them. But if you want to strengthen an element, you need to do the meridian exercises of the corresponding element on a daily basis for a minimum of three weeks. After the three weeks, evaluate the effect these exercises are having on your body and on your mental and emotional life. Then decide whether to do the exercises daily for three months. If you do the following exercises on a regular basis, you will increasingly experience the strength of Wood in your body and in your actions; you will feel fitter and more decisive, and your vision will probably improve.

For each organ, two exercises are described. They strengthen the flow of *Qi* through the organ and its corresponding meridian. Thus, they enhance the physiological, emotional, mental, and spiritual functions of the organ. The first exercise consists of a physical posture combined with a visualization of the corresponding meridian. This exercise also helps you to develop a feeling for the quality of the corresponding organ and element. The second exercise directly activates the flow of *Qi* in the actual meridian.

STRENGTHENING THE WOOD-YANG: THE GALL BLADDER POSTURE   The posture shown in the photograph depicts the essence of the Chinese understanding of the Gall Bladder. It represents the spirit of beginning, setting out on something new, making a decision, and being driven. It depicts life as "the way," and the significance of traveling actively along that path.

This posture will introduce you to the flow of the Gall Bladder Meridian. Imagine a red or orange energy river about two inches wide that begins at your right eye and flows downward to your feet; this is the meridian. Strengthen the image in your imagination with every exhalation.

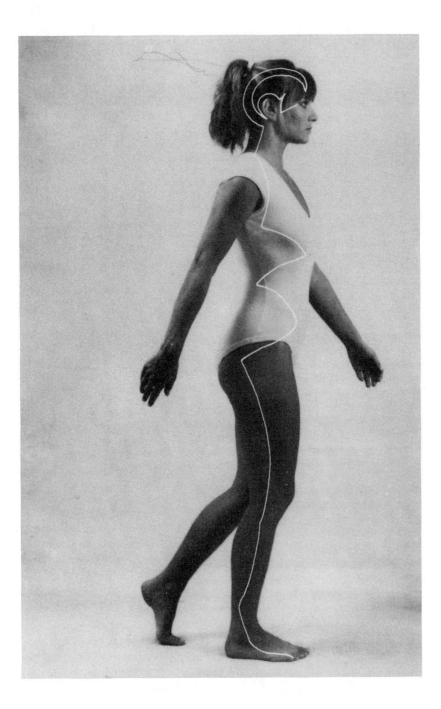

Mental and Physical Exercises to Stimulate the Growth of Wood

Then begin to walk slowly back and forth, continuing to concentrate on the flow of the meridian. After two or three minutes, repeat the exercise visualizing the Gall Bladder Meridian on your left side.

Activating the Gall Bladder Meridian

1. Stand with your feet parallel, spread a couple of feet apart. Your shoulders should be relaxed, arms hanging loosely at your sides. Your knees should be slightly bent.
2. Extend your arms straight above your head, with the palms of your hands facing each other.
3. Inhaling, bend your body as far to the left as you can. Your arms should remain as straight as possible. As you stretch to the side, keep your torso aligned and look straight ahead. Let the weight of your right arm stretch your right side so that you have the feeling of a taught bow extending down into your right foot.
4. Stand up straight again. Exhale intensely and, with your hands made into fists, move in one sudden movement into a stooped position with your knees slighty bent.
5. As you inhale, stand up straight and repeat the exercise, this time bending to the right.
6. Repeat this exercise 10 times on each side.

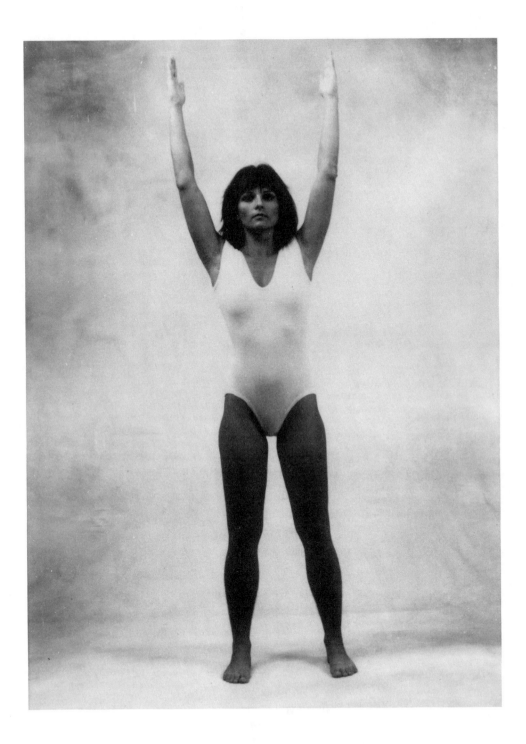

Mental and Physical Exercises to Stimulate the Growth of Wood

STRENGTHENING THE WOOD-YIN: THE LIVER POSTURE   This posture embodies the essence of the Liver energy: the tree, physical growth, balance, coordinated strength, and quiet concentration on the essential.

Visualize your Liver Meridian as a river of energy that flows from your big toe up to your chest. Strengthen your visualization of this flow with every inhalation. Stay in this posture for at least a minute. Then repeat the exercise with the other leg. If you have difficulty maintaining your balance, it is a sign that you are not rooted enough in yourself.

Activating the Liver Meridian

1. Lie on your back and bring your ankles toward your buttocks so that your knees are bent and pointing to the ceiling. Hold your ankles with your hands. Your feet should be flat on the floor.
2. Breathe in while raising your hips as high as possible from the ground, and breathe out while lowering your body back to the floor.

Mental and Physical Exercises to Stimulate the Growth of Wood

3. Repeat this exercise for a minute. Then lift your hips one last time as high as possible and remain in this position. At the same time, tighten your buttocks and stomach muscles as much as possible. Then let yourself sink back into a state of relaxation.

4. Lie flat on your back with your eyes closed and be aware of your body.

part 3

火

FIRE

The Element Fire

THE power of Fire manifests itself in the afternoon and in the south, in warmth, in the blooming of flowers, and in the summer. Fire follows Wood in the *Sheng* cycle; wood is used to make fire (see Part VII, The Four Cycles later in this book). Fire is called the "old Yang." Fire is the only element that is embodied in four organs: in the Heart, the Small Intestine, the Pericardium or Heart Governor, and the Triple Warmer. Fire manifests itself in our tongue and speech. It governs the blood vessels: the capillaries, arteries, and veins. Its bodily fluid is perspiration.

The nature of Wood is expansion, growth in all directions. The power of Fire is directed vertically upward, from deep in the earth up into the sky, from the material to the spiritual, from unawareness to consciousness, in the opposite direction of gravity. On the mental-emotional level, Fire brings out joy, dancing, laughter, awareness, and the ability to have an encompassing view of things. Its colors are scarlet and red.

Ancient China had a court culture with a strict hierarchy. The social order, which was centered around the Emperor and his royal household, was thought to be responsible for maintaining harmony between heaven and earth. In contrast to Greek philosophy (which emerges from the cosmos and the laws of nature) and the Indian philosophy of the *Vedas* and the *Upanishads* (which recognizes the inner self as the essence of the universe), Chinese cosmology finds its central themes in the order of society and ethics: correct personal behavior brings forth the proper behavior of nature. If society, especially the Emperor and his court members in the center, followed the laws of the *Tao*, then the land would be spared hardships, including floods, droughts, epidemics, hunger, and typhoons. This social-mystical viewpoint held the society together.

This belief also permeated Chinese medicine, in that the human body was seen as the court, and the different organs as the civil servants. If individuals fulfilled their social responsibilities, honored their ancestors, placated their demons, and maintained contact with the Elements operating through their organs, thoughts, and actions, then illnesses stayed away from them.

The first Yin organ of Fire is the Heart. It is called the Fire Prince, the highest ruler of the organs. It is seen as the center of consciousness, feelings, and thoughts. Yin *Shen*, the spirit of Fire, rules the heart. The Chinese character *Shen* can be translated as "spirit," "soul," "God," "godly," and "effectiveness." The meaning of this character is touched upon when one says that a person has spirit.

Shen has two houses. The lower residence is the heart, where it ensures balanced feelings and a clear, honest way of speaking. Its higher house is the third eye, or forehead *chakra* (a Hindu term for energy center), where it brings forth clarity of thoughts and a conscious life direction. When these characteristics are present in a person, that person's *Shen* is powerful and healthy. One recognizes this as a sparkle or light in the eyes.

If, however, *Shen* is confused or lacking in energy, it is noticeable in unclear thinking or an inability to organize thoughts; in speech defects ranging from lisping, stammering, or stuttering to muteness; or in emotions full of highs and lows, one minute shouting for joy, the next minute wanting to die. This includes different forms of hysteria and manic depression. A dispersed, confused *Shen* expresses itself in nervousness, fearfulness, stage fright, insomnia, and dull, unfocused eyes. All of these symptoms are caused by a disturbance in the Fire element.

When the Fire energy in the heart is too strong, the Chinese say it is *Shi*, in excess. This results in talkativeness, excessive perspiration, and nervous tension. People with this condition believe that they have to take everything into their own hands; they must control everything. Most of the time they are not capable of letting other people take responsibility. This is a characteristic of contemporary "manager sickness," which often leads to heart failure. The "Type A" personality and its stress-related illnesses, characterized by high blood pressure and heart attacks, are manifestations of *Shi* in the heart. As we will see later, this imbalance typically emerges as a result of an energy deficit in the Water element.

When the Fire energy in the heart is too weak, it is called *Xu*, deficient. This leads to disturbances such as inability to express oneself clearly, partial or total muteness, and a dulled or nonfunctioning sense of taste, both on the tongue and in the psyche.

The second Yin organ of Fire is the Pericardium, also called the Heart Cover or Heart Governor. It is designated in the Chinese tradition as the first minister or chancellor of the Fire Prince, as bodyguard and protector of the heart, as its castle. Its task is to protect the prince from harm and defeat, to give orders to the court officials and subjects, and to report to the prince about his well-being. In people, it brings about the ability to be generous to oneself and to others, to radiate warmth, and to love. The Heart Governor expresses itself in the ability to give and in the ability to accept complaints, lamentations, criticism, and love from others. When this characteristic is developed, a person is able to speak from the heart and be cordial and affectionate, enthusiastic, humorous, and hearty. In contrast, we speak of some people as being cold-hearted or small-minded, as if they have a heart of stone. A serious form of inflammation of the Pericardium can lead to a so-called "armored heart" on an organic level.

In Chinese physiology, the duties of the Heart and the Pericardium also include the maintenance and regulation of the circulatory system. Accordingly, the arteries and veins are categorized as the "tissue" of Fire. The Heart, Pericardium, blood vessels, and all of the hormones and regulatory mechanisms having to do with the maintenance and control of the circulatory system through dilation or contraction of the blood vessels form a functional unit.

In ancient Chinese texts, the Pericardium is spoken of as the Yang-Kidney. In modern Chinese medicine, the term "Yang-Kidney" refers to the suprarenal glands, whose main function, besides regulating the metabolism, is to control the circulatory system and the fluid and electrolyte levels. This means that, in ancient times, the Pericardium was thought of as pertaining to the Water element, whereas, in this century, the Pericardium is considered the second Fire-Yin organ. But it is important to remember that the functions of the Yang-Kidney and the Pericardium are closely linked, and that the Pericardium occupies a central position between the Kidney and the Heart, between Water and Fire, between the upper and lower poles of a person.

To further understand this, it should be noted that the Chinese recognize six different energy layers in the human organism, each layer being nourished, maintained, and regulated by two organs. The innermost layer, the core of our body and personality, is made up of the Kidney and the Heart. These two organs build our vertical axis, our basic polarity of *Hara* and head. Heart and Kidney form the polarity of Fire and Water, of above and below, of Heaven and Earth, of God and the Devil, of Zeus and Hades, Jupiter and Pluto.

In India, the worship of Shiva, the destroyer, is placed on the same level as those of Brahma, the creator, and Vishnu, the maintainer. In China, the balance between above and below, and right and left, is seen as desirable. However, in Western civilization, a higher value is placed on the upper pole. This belief has led to a one-sided effort—a striving that is directed "above," to the "good," "to get into heaven"—and with that, to the creation of evil and our concept of hell. In Western cultures, the areas of Fire—love, speech, and intellect—are more treasured than the depths of Water—sexuality, meditation, and sinking into the archaic levels of the soul. Just think of the beginning of the Gospel according to John: "In the beginning was the word, and the word was with God, and God was the word. And the word became flesh and dwelled among us."

If the Pericardium is in balance, it forms a bridge between Water and Fire, and we experience a fulfilled sexuality that brings forth joy and laughter. If the *Qi* flows in the Pericardium, we feel a deep connection between sexual lust and love, and we are able to freely give and receive. During the seventies, in an attempt to free sexuality from damnation, our culture paid much more attention to the physical orgasm, which is a function of the Water element, than to the needs of the soul. Only in the eighties—in part due to the advent of AIDS—did the union of Water and Fire in love and sexuality become more important again.

Although the Heart and Pericardium are two Yin organs belonging to the same element, they have vastly different tasks. The heart is responsible for "inner matters." Its functions include clarity of thought, speech, responsibility, and motivation. This is also expressed in the names of a few of the points on the Heart Meridian. *Shenmen* (Heart 7) means "Gate of the Spirit" or "Gate of the Consciousness." *Tongli* (Heart 5) means "Relationship to the Inner." On the other hand, the Pericardium is responsible for "outer matters," regulating blood circulation, heartbeat, and heart frequency on the organic level. Cold hands and feet are a symptom of a lack of energy in the Pericardium. A person with little warmth has an energy deficit in the Pericardium. This includes people who do not find much joy in sexuality, stingy people who have a difficult time giving, people who need a long time to thaw, and closed people who don't laugh.

Because of this, points on the Heart Meridian are usually used in treating psychological disorders, for example insomnia, nervousness, hysteria, manic depression, and epilepsy. They are also used to treat speech disorders and people who have difficulty listening to others. However, the points on the Pericardium Meridian are more likely to help when there is a physical problem with the heart, for example heart pains, angina pectoris, tachycardia, heartbeat irregularities, or circulatory problems. But, of course, points on the Pericardium channel also have a marked psychological effect.

The Small Intestine is the Yang organ assigned to the Heart. The key to understanding its function is seen in the assimilation of nourishment in the digestive process. Just as the Small Intestine takes care that nourishment can be absorbed in the blood, it is also responsible on an intellectual level for the assimilation of ideas. An energy deficit in the Small Intestine is manifested in a person who takes on knowledge, convictions, and beliefs from others undigested, and is not capable of developing personal views and belief systems out of this. The appearance of a person who is able to assimilate is displayed through a fine, silent laughing in the eyes and around the lips.

The Triple Warmer, or *Sanjiao*, is the second Yang organ of Fire; it is assigned to the Pericardium. The Triple Warmer is an association of various functions in the body and mind, rather than an organic reality. The Chinese teachings speak of the *Sanjiao* as the "three burning cavities" in the organism: the chest (for breathing), the abdomen (for digestion), and the pelvis (for excretion and reproduction). The task of the Triple Warmer is to coordinate these three areas of the body, for instance coordinating the depth and frequency of breath in relation to digestion and sexuality, and regulating body temperature and equilibrium. It is assumed that the Chinese term *Sanjiao* also includes the different centers for the regulation of body temperature in the brain, especially the hypothalamus.

The Triple Warmer is the most complex of the organs, and because of this it is also the easiest to bring out of balance in the entire organism. In classical texts, it appears as the foreign minister of Fire, the protector of the Yin and Yang organs, the energy minister who oversees the production of the different types of *Qi* and guarantees its distribution in the body.

When the Fire element in a person is balanced, summer brings joy and fulfillment. Such people have an inner balance from which to oversee events. They know when to speak and when to remain silent. They can feel joy without becoming excessive. They can steer and lead others, but they know when the time is right to pull back. Their eyes glow. They know goodness and magnanimity, and they have good taste.

Mental and Physical Exercises to Ignite the Fire

CLARIFYING QUESTIONS

Ask yourself the following questions as you have done with Wood:

- How do I feel in summer, in the heat, or in the south?
- Do I perspire easily?
- Do I talk too much or too little?
- Can I satisfyingly communicate my needs and ideas?
- Can I react spontaneously to an unforeseen and unexpected situation?
- Do I listen attentively to others, or do I think about what I want to say while they are still talking?
- When was the last time I laughed heartily?
- In what situations do I have no sense of humor?
- Do others sometimes judge me as being arrogant, haughty, and proud?
- Do others perceive me as adamant, hard-hearted, and cruel?
- Do I often have cold hands and feet?
- Do I take my duties very, very seriously?
- Am I ready to trust other people with important tasks and decisions?
- Do I sleep deeply, or do I have insomnia?

- How healthy is my heart?
- Am I clear about what is most important to me in life?
- Do I try very hard to always direct what is happening around me?
- Am I sometimes as happy as a small child?
- Who do I love?
- Making love, do I sometimes feel a deep joy?
- Do I sometimes start laughing out of joy while making love?
- Do other people sometimes tell me that my eyes have a sparkle, a shine, a brilliance?

FIRE EXERCISES

LOOKING INTO THE FIRE   Go into the forest in the afternoon, gather wood, and make a campfire. Sit on the north side of the fire facing the south, so that you are looking into the fire. Direct your attention effortlessly and continuously into the flames until you sense that your thoughts have become slower and your consciousness has become filled with the fire. While you are doing this, you can imagine that your thoughts are being devoured by the flames and that your intellect has become one single flame.

Enjoy this state of being for about 15 minutes.

LIGHT MEDITATION   This technique is useful for bringing your mind to rest.

Place a burning candle two to three feet away from you. Look into the flame without blinking. Relax your eyes and sink into a state as I have described above.

Do this exercise once a day for two to three weeks if you want to feel an effect on your life.

MIRROR MEDITATION   Sit comfortably in front of a mirror and look into your eyes for at least half an hour. Allow your focus to be soft so that you can see your entire face. After a while, you will see other faces and images emerge from under the surface of your own trusted face. This is especially likely to happen if you do this meditation at sundown or in candlelight.

You can also do this exercise with a partner. Sit across from each other, about five feet apart, and look into each other's eyes for at least half an hour. You can do this exercise with someone you love; it can also be helpful when you've had a fight in which discussion no longer helps.

EXERCISES FOR THE MERIDIANS OF THE HEART, SMALL INTESTINE, PERICARDIUM, AND SANJIAO

STRENGTHENING THE FIRE-YIN: THE HEART POSTURE This posture speaks for itself. It shows grace and surrender, simplicity and clarity, the ability to be a king as well as a servant.

Enter this posture when you are confused, when disorder reigns in your life, or when you catch yourself under constant stress and have no idea why you don't trust anyone to help you.

Visualize the Heart Meridian, which runs from the middle of the underarm to the inside of the little finger. Intensify your image of this

Mental and Physical Exercises to Ignite the Fire

energy flow in your thoughts each time you exhale. Hold this posture for at least three minutes.

Activating the Heart Meridian

1. Stand with your feet parallel, two foot lengths apart. Hold both arms bent, shoulders relaxed, with the palms of your hands facing upward.
2. Make loose fists.
3. Imagine a reservoir of energy (*Qi*) just below your navel; this point is called the *Hara*.
4. Imagine that, with each exhalation, the *Qi* penetrates into your left fist, and move your fist horizontally forward, as if to punch something. Carry out this movement slowly.
5. With the next inhalation, pull your fist slowly back to its original position.
6. Make the same movement with your right arm.
7. While exhaling, slowly stretch your left fist horizontally to the side. While inhaling, bring it back to its original position.
8. Do the same with your right arm.
9. Repeat this sequence at least five times. When exhaling, imagine that the *Qi* is bringing about the movement, and, when inhaling, that the *Qi* is returning to the *Hara* (the pelvis).

Mental and Physical Exercises to Ignite the Fire

55

THE PERICARDIUM POSTURE   This posture embodies the essence of the Pericardium: openness, warmth, the willingness to give, and the willingness to receive from others. This posture can help you to develop these characteristics.

When you take this posture, visualize the meridian shown in the picture. It flows from the heart to the hand: It flows one inch away from the sides of the nipples along the surface of the body and runs along the insides of the arms to the last joint of the middle finger. Intensify the energy flow in your imagination while you exhale. Remain in this posture until your hands feel warm and charged.

Chinese Medicine for Beginners

Activating the Pericardium

1. Sit on the floor and bring the soles of your feet together.
2. Rest your hands under your feet with the palms facing up, so that the outsides of your ankles are lying on your hands. The point in the middle of the inside of the wrist is Pericardium 7, The Source. It is stimulated through this exercise.
3. While you exhale, stretch the upper part of your body gently in the direction of your feet. While you inhale, return to the original position. Do this exercise for one minute, then remain sitting quietly in this position with your eyes closed and experience the effects of this exercise.

Mental and Physical Exercises to Ignite the Fire

STRENGTHENING THE FIRE-YANG: THE POSTURE OF THE SMALL INTESTINE This posture is that of a Kung-Fu fighter using the *Qi* energy won through assimilation in the small intestine for his self-defense. "The organs, small intestine, and bladder eat the *Tai Yang*, the highest Yang, an energy which protects the body from without."

Take the position of the fighter. Tighten your body like a wound-up spring, holding your arm stretched out in front of you. Imagine the Small Intestine Meridian on your right side: the energy flows through this meridian from the tip of your little finger, over your shoulder blade, to your ear. Intensify this flow in your imagination while you inhale. Stay in this posture until you become warm or hot. Then do the exercise on your left side.

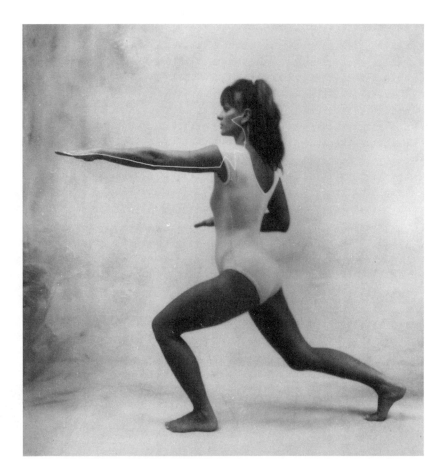

Chinese Medicine for Beginners

Activating the Small Intestine Meridian

1. Sit on your heels and bring your forehead to the ground. Clasp your hands together behind your back, palms turned toward each other.

2. Inhale and stretch your arms upward and forward, so that you feel the tension in your shoulders and shoulder blades. Remain in this posture for about 30 seconds, breathing deeply through your nose.

3. Then stretch your arms a bit farther forward until the tension climaxes.

4. Exhale and let your arms relax on the ground. Feel the effects of this exercise on your body.

Mental and Physical Exercises to Ignite the Fire

STRENGTHENING THE SECOND FIRE-YANG: THE *SANJIAO* POSTURE

This posture is that of a bird in flight. It expresses the essence of the Triple Warmer: the coordination of the chest, abdomen, and pelvis—of breathing, digestion, and sexuality.

Take the posture of the flying bird and breathe fully and deeply through your mouth. Breathe into your chest and abdomen. Hold your arms stretched out and your head tilted slightly to the side. Visualize the Meridian of the Triple Warmer on your right side, which runs from the ring finger along the arm to the ear, and then to the outside of the eyebrow. Remain in this pose until you become warm or hot. Be careful to remain loose, and do not become cramped. Then do the exercise on the left side.

Chinese Medicine for Beginners

Activating the Sanjaio

1. Sit on the ground with your legs stretched out in front of you. Rest your hands behind you on the ground with your fingertips pointing away from you.
2. Raise your pelvis so that your body forms a straight line from your head to your toes.
3. Breathe deeply and regularly for about one minute.
4. Stretch yourself out on the ground keeping your eyes closed, and relax into the pleasant, warm sensation that is created by this exercise.

Mental and Physical Exercises to Ignite the Fire

part 4

EARTH

The Element Earth

THE season of the year for Earth is late summer, the time when the sun is in the zodiac sign of Virgo. It is the time when nature displays warmth, fullness, and abundance. It is the time when the grains are harvested, and the time of harvest festivals. In farming communities, the fruits of the forest and fields are gathered, sorted out, and dried, and the storage cellars and pantries are filled. An important task during this time of year is the choosing and preparation of foodstuffs that will ensure survival in winter. It is necessary to be concerned that the provisions last for the whole winter. It is the time of gathering and of collecting, as the climax of summer with its dance festivals, love affairs, and pleasures is over, and what is left behind are the nostalgic memories of what was experienced. While in spring a person looks forward to summer, and in summer experiences the pleasures of the present moment, late summer is the time to look back at what was and process it.

The middle is the direction assigned to Earth; it is neither Yin nor Yang; the direction of its energy is a horizontal, closed circle. Late summer is the time when nature makes the transition from its Yang phase to its Yin phase. In spring and summer, the powers of light prevail and all the manifestations of nature spread themselves out, grow higher, and turn themselves to the sky and the sun. In fall and winter, the powers of darkness prevail. Nature hides; it draws back inside itself.

The transition periods between the seasons are also assigned to the element Earth. These are moments for looking inside and collecting oneself before a new phase begins.

The colors of Earth are yellow and brown; its climate is moist, as, without water and dampness, the fullness and fertility of the earth cannot manifest themselves. For Europeans, this allocation does not seem to be very important, as there is enough moisture throughout the year at this latitude. However, in the tropics and subtropics—and large parts of China fall within this area—late summer is the time of the monsoon with its fierce, gushing rainfall and its steamy humidity that follows the glaring heat of the summer and makes the earth fertile again.

In almost all myths, the earth plays an important role. The fertility goddesses and earth goddesses are one symbol in most cultures, bringing the earth, motherliness, and the sustaining of life together with security and safety, nourishment and fertility, and fullness and generosity. In people, Earth expresses itself through compassion, recognition, sympathy, and a feeling of love and unity with one's environment—through a basic feeling that one is welcome and at home where one is at that moment.

One also finds this feeling in people who quickly gain a sense of well-being in a new environment and who feel accepted by others. This basic feeling gives self-assurance that doesn't need to be proven, an inner security and calmness. In contrast to this, people with a weakness in the Earth element feel insecure, often begging for attention and affection. Underneath this behavior lies the fear that warmth and affection could be taken away or denied. This attitude is often found in people who were not nourished with much love in their early childhood, or who often had to change residences or familiar environments. In psychotherapy today, this behavioral complex is called an "oral fixation."

People with an imbalance in the element Earth often lack compassion; they seem not to enter into relationships with others, and the affairs of others don't seem to touch them very much. A critical stance toward others usually goes hand in hand with this, wherein harsh judgments and low tolerance mask one's own insecurity. With the help of critical remarks, these people are trying to build up their own sense of superiority. Another manifestation of a weakened Earth is self-pity and a constant whining about one's own problems. Such people often play the martyr. A classical example of this is the woman who sacrifices herself for her husband and children, not treating herself to anything. She can moan and point to her destiny as the reason for this.

The search for missing security is the driving force and main occupation of people with weak Earth. They look for this security in eating or in smoking, or they are overly affectionate, grasping for love, and constantly looking for the security of motherly love in their relationships. They often hide their fear of abandonment behind a romantic ideal of love and partnership.

A person with a healthy Earth element has an inner abundance from which to give and care for others. Such a person has a sweet scent, just as most fruits have a sweet scent and flavor in late summer when nature displays fullness and abundance. If, however, the Earth element is lacking, it leads to a constant overflow of sticky emotional outbursts and to over-exaggerated generosity, which serves to make others dependent. This behavior is often found in mothers who hinder their children from becoming adults by limiting their responsibilities and not allowing them to make decisions. The tender, lightly sweet scent of the earth becomes unpleasantly sweet in such people. The natural desire for ripe fruits and grains becomes an addiction to sweet things. The melodic, singing quality that the earth gives to the voice becomes a whining, moaning sing-song.

Only where there is inner security is there a purpose for oneself, and a reality in which fullness and abundance are possible. Only when possessing this fullness is a person able to love and care for others. Without this inner wealth, the pleasant, sweet quality of the earth turns into an outer show—a mask covering one's own emptiness.

The elemental spirit of Earth is called *Yi*. Its homes are the spleen and pancreas, the Yin organs of Earth. Its qualities are logical thinking and a rational intellect, the ability to be critical, the ability to think things over, and a good memory. Other characteristics are worrying about a thousand and one things or brooding over the past and indulging in reminiscences. On a mental level, the effect of Earth can be seen in the same concepts and categories that are used to label the period of late summer: gathering, processing, selecting, mental nourishment, survival, and gaining the wisdom that gives us the security to deal with difficult situations in life.

The word "intellect" comes from the Latin verb *legere,* which means "to read" and "to gather." An intellectual reads a lot, broods over things, gathers information in the brain, stores it, and processes it—if the intellect has enough Fire, enough independence, to be able to digest and assimilate the gathered ideas.

The greed for knowledge and the latest news, and an addiction to reading, can be traced to an overstimulated spleen. Above all, this is displayed in an accumulation of knowledge about detailed areas of human life—in the type of knowledge that specialists have, concentrated without seeing the connection to the bigger picture.

A *Shi* state, or Fullness, of the spleen is also found in people who cannot stop thinking—who have to think through and consider everything, whose intellect is constantly caught in an inner monologue. A *Shi* state of the spleen can also be found in one-sided advocates of science and reason, in people who judge and reject every other way of looking at things. Such people try to compensate for a deficit in Earth energy by mentally clinging to an apparent security in the logical verification of things.

Other symptoms of a *Shi* state of the spleen are compulsive behavior, fixed ideas, obsessions, and a passion for collecting. If the person is a collector, the degree of imbalance can be recognized in whether that person gathers useful and valuable objects—for example, paintings or antiques—or completely absurd objects that have become an obsession.

One can also see different forms and levels of obsession. In our culture, many people are obsessed with an idea or a way of life: work, status, power, success, and money. In ancient China, one spoke more commonly of an obsession in relation to being possessed by demons and spirits, although it is actually the same phenomenon: an idea or a demon gets the upper hand in a person's mind to such an extent that this person becomes blind to the variety of life, losing contact with the body, feelings, and self.

All people have an individually varying supply of elemental energies available to express themselves on the physical, emotional, and mental levels. For instance, if a person uses up a large portion of Earth energy for taking in nourishment and digestion, there won't be much energy left over for thought and reflection. If a person uses up a large portion of Earth energy through intellectual work, there will be a deficit on the organic and emotional levels. Such a person will have little compassion because the intellect is so occupied with other things. And if you use up a lot of your Earth energy through your thinking process, there will probably be a deficit of Earth energy on the physical level sooner or later, leading to allergies, or menstrual problems, or stomach ulcers and metabolic disorders.

The Yin organ of Earth is commonly called the Spleen. As I mentioned in the chapter on the organs, Chinese medicine has a more energetic approach to the body, and that is why organs are defined in a different way. On the physical level, the Spleen consists of two main systems or "organs" in the body: first, the exocrinic part of the pancreas and, second, the Reticulo-Endothelial System (RES), a network of reticular connective tissue and endothelium that forms various anatomical structures in the body.

The exocrinic part of the pancreas produces preliminary digestive enzymes that enter the digestive tract in the middle of the duodenum. Their function is to break down proteins, fats, and carbohydrates. They become highly activated in the duodenum and small intestine, where they finish the digestive process begun in the mouth and stomach.

In the Chinese tradition, the duodemun and the first six inches of the small intestine are considered part of the stomach. This is important because a large part of the absorption of nutrients takes place in the first six inches of the small intestine. Consequently, one can understand why the Chinese attribute the digestion of food and nourishment of the body to the Earth organs and, only to a lesser extent, to the small intestine.

"RES" is a medical term that describes, on one hand, the lymphatic tissues and organs: the spleen, lymph nodes, lymphatic vessels, tonsils, appendix, and thymus. On the other hand, the RES also includes the red bone marrow, the copper star cells of the liver, and the mucus membranes of the intestine with its large number of lymph follicles.

The major tasks of the lymphatic system can be summarized as follows:

1. Draining: the transport of "excess" water from the tissue back into the blood;
2. Absorption of fat from the intestine to the intestinal lymphatic vessels;
3. Generation of lymphocytes (the essential part of the body's immune system) in the bone marrow, lymph nodes, and spleen;
4. Storage and breakdown of red blood cells in the spleen.

If one ties together the above descriptions of the functions of the pancreas and RES, one can see a clear picture of the functions of the Earth organs according to the traditional view. The Spleen is the mother organ of the physical body. The Spleen regulates the distribution of water and blood. It is the nourisher of the body. The organic tissues that are assigned to Earth are the connective tissue, fat tissue, and muscle fibers. The Spleen's Yang organ is the Stomach, and its sensory organ the mouth, especially the lips and the mouth cavity. It communicates to the outer world through taste and touch. Its bodily fluids are saliva and lymph.

The main function of the Earth organs is nourishment and maintenance of the body. In contrast to our understanding, the Chinese notion of "nourishment" refers not only to providing nutrients, but also to providing oxygen via the erythrocytes to every cell in the body. The erythrocytes—or red blood cells—are formed in the red bone marrow that belongs to the Spleen. That is why the ancient texts emphasized: "The Spleen regulates the blood."

Another important aspect of maintaining the body's integrity is the work of the immune system, whose components belong to the Spleen. The red bone marrow generates the B-lymphocytes, which produce antibodies; the lymphatic organs (primarily the lymph glands and the spleen) generate the T-lymphocytes, which are programmed to fight specific antigens.

As the lymphatic vessels transport fluids from the tissue to the blood stream, the Spleen regulates the distribution of water in the body in general, and especially the tone of the skin. As long as our Spleen is vital and strong, we radiate youth and health.

Because the Earth organs nourish and maintain the body, the Spleen is seen not only as the mother of the physical body, but also as the organ responsible for fertility, pregnancy, and birth, in conjunction with the Kidney and the Uterus. The breasts are assigned to the element Earth, whereas the Uterus is considered an extraordinary organ.

Out of this composition, the clinical meaning of the Spleen and Stomach Meridians becomes clear. An imbalance results in disorders including illnesses of the digestive system such as indigestion, gastritis, stomach and duodenum ulcers, incomplete digestion, pancreatitis, diarrhea, and constipation; illnesses of the immune system such as allergies, autoimmune diseases (in which Wood also plays a part), immune deficiencies, a disposition toward illness, menstrual problems, infertility, pain and swelling of the breasts (especially in connection with the menses), inflammation of the mammary glands, problems with lactating, skin diseases, edema, and swelling; and, finally, illnesses of the lymph nodes and lymphatic vessels.

Disturbances in the rhythm of the human organism point to an imbalance in the element Earth. The rhythms of sleeping and waking, of appetite and digestion, and of breathing, as well as the menstrual cycle and the rhythm of physical, spiritual, and mental activity, are all determined by the revolution of the earth on its axis. They follow the rhythm of day and night, the cycle of the moon and the tides, and the changing of the seasons. Because the moon is so closely connected to the rhythms of the earth, in many cultures it is assigned to Earth and is seen as the symbol for fertility and birth. However, it is also often assigned to Water, as its revolution affects the tides. The Earth plays a central role in the Chinese way of thinking. In the original diagrams of the five elements, Earth is portrayed in the center, and the elements Water, Wood, Fire, and Metal and the four directions arrange themselves around it. In ancient China, there were medical and spiritual schools based on handling every physical and spiritual complaint by bringing the element Earth into balance. They attained this through an extensive, practical knowledge about the powers of the elements in various foods, through the use of herbs and extracts of herbs, through massage and acupuncture of the stomach and spleen-pancreas meridians, and through special mental and physical exercises to strengthen the Earth energy in a person's disposition.

Our language includes many ways to express our connection with Earth: "standing with both feet on the ground," "mother earth," "to not feel the ground under one's feet," and many more. The earth is our central, physical reality from the moment we begin our lives in the womb until we return to the earth. Our sense of reality is based on the strength of the Earth element in us. How we present ourselves, whether we have both feet on the ground, whether we feel "at home" and secure in our lives, whether we feel comfortable in our skin, and whether we radiate and look healthy and vital all depend on our connection to Earth.

Mental and Physical Exercises to Strengthen the Earth

CLARIFYING QUESTIONS

Proceed with the questions as you have done previously.

- Do I feel comfortable in my surroundings most of the time?
- Do I feel comfortable in my skin?
- Do I generally feel loved and accepted by the people around me, or do I feel unloved and misunderstood?
- Do I get the attention I want?
- Am I a compassionate person?
- Do other people come to me to tell me their worries and problems, or am I occupied most of the time with my own affairs?
- Am I more likely to be good-natured or demanding?
- Am I possessive in a love relationship?
- Do I have a rigid idea of how my relationship with my partner should be?
- Do I try to control my partner or to change his or her ways?
- Can I be happy about how my partner is?
- Do I have a strong, healthy constitution, or am I often sick?

- Do I suffer from allergies?
- Do I sleep deeply and have a healthy appetite and a glowing appearance?
- Do I like to eat, and do I take pleasure in it?
- Do I have a healthy stomach?
- Am I preoccupied with my diet, eating habits, and nourishment ideals?
- Do I eat my meals with regularity?
- Do I sometimes have a feeling of fullness in my abdomen after I eat?
- Do I have a firm or a flabby body?
- Am I overly critical of myself or others?

EARTH EXERCISES

GROUNDING YOURSELF   It is best to do this exercise in the forest, on a lawn, or on the beach. However, it can also be done on a blanket in your room. A good time for this exercise is in the afternoon or early evening.

Lie on your stomach and stretch yourself out like a cat. Then let yourself sink into the ground. Imagine that you are composed of earth—heavy and still.

Remain in this position for at least 15 minutes. To concentrate your thoughts, use the mantra "*Yi.*" If you want to strengthen the power in your *Hara*, place a tennis ball underneath your abdomen, about two finger-widths below your belly button. With every breath, relax your abdomen more and more.

COMPASSION   Look for someone around you who needs attention. Take two hours of your time to be with him or her. Find out what this person needs and what makes him or her happy.

EATING CONSCIOUSLY   Prepare your own meals for a week. Prepare food that tastes good, is easy to digest, and gives you strength. Enjoy it! Invite someone to eat with you occasionally.

Exercises for the Stomach and Spleen Meridians

Strengthening the Earth-Yang: The Stomach Posture This posture represents the circle—the circle being the symbol of earth.

Hold this posture for a minute. Breathe regularly through your mouth, which should be slightly open. Make sure that the palm of your upper hand is facing the ceiling, and that the palm of your lower hand is facing the ground. Visualize the Stomach Meridian first only on the right side, on the side of your raised arm. The energy flows through the meridian from a point under your right eye, down your face and neck, to the middle of your right clavicle. From there, the meridian runs down across the chest to your right nipple, and further down over the abdomen to the pubic bone. There, the meridian crosses the groin to the outside and runs along the front of the leg, down to the tip of the second toe. Imagine a yellow stream of energy that runs down this meridian and into the ground, helping you to feel the ground underneath your feet more intensely.

After a minute, exhale and stretch your right hand as far up as you can and your left hand as far down as you can. Then take the posture for the left side and visualize the left Stomach Meridian.

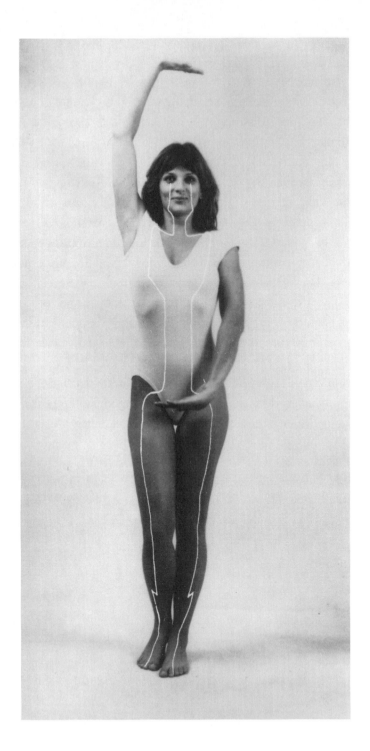

Activating the Stomach Meridian

Sit on the ground with your legs bent under you so that your feet are on either side of your hips. Lower the upper part of your body slowly backward until you feel a tension in your thighs. If you are able, lie for half a minute with your back on the ground and breathe deeply in and out.

Mental and Physical Exercises to Strengthen the Earth

STRENGTHENING THE EARTH-YIN: THE SPLEEN POSTURE   This posture expresses security, being grounded, and stability—essential qualities of the Spleen energy.

Hold this posture for at least a minute. The distance between your feet should be great enough to allow you to easily let your pelvis sink down. Breathe regularly through your mouth, which should be slightly open. Slowly turn your torso to the right, then to the left, then again to the right, and so on.

The *Qi* flows through this meridian from the big toe, up the inside of the leg to the groin and to the abdomen, from there further to the breast, and to just before the armpit. Then the meridian runs a bit farther down to its endpoint, which is in the middle of the flank. Imagine that you pull the *Qi* up through the meridian to its endpoint with every inhalation.

While you turn your torso to the right, visualize the left Spleen Meridian with every inhalation. While you exhale, turn your torso back to its original position. While you are turning to the left, visualize the right Spleen Meridian with every inhalation.

Activating the Spleen Meridian

1. Lie on your stomach with your hands underneath your body so that your fists are under your groin.

2. Breathe in and raise your stretched legs as far as possible off the ground. Remain in this position for half a minute, breathing deeply in and out.

3. While breathing out, lower your legs slowly to the ground and let your arms relax next to your body. Be careful that no tension remains in the small of your back.

4. Lie for another minute on your stomach and imagine that your body is filled with the color yellow.

part 5

METAL

The Element Metal

FALL depicts the essence of Metal: concentration and condensation; the energy is directed within. The withering of plants and the withdrawal of the life force that we experience in fall is the exact opposite of the expansive energy of spring. Metal is the opposite of Wood. Just as Wood is called the "young Yang," Metal embodies the "young Yin." Its direction is the west; its climate dry; its time of day evening.

The four elements of Western tradition are earth, air, fire, and water. In ancient Greek culture, there was originally a fifth element—spirit or ether—whose characteristics are found not only in Wood and Fire, but also in Metal. Metal corresponds to the Greek element of air, although it has additional meanings. The names of some points on the Lung Meridian show the relationship to air—for example Lung 2, "The Gate to the Clouds," and Lung 3, "Palace of Heaven"—but the meanings of most of the names go deeper, as the essence of the element Metal is structure, distance, depth, and dimension. This expresses itself in names such as "Large Abyss" (Lu 9), "Missing Order" (Lu 7), and "Oblique Junction" (LI 6).

Metal symbolizes concentrated energy, an essence that keeps the universe together. Power spots in nature were used by ancient cultures for ritual purposes. They built their temples and churches and even magnificent structures such as the Cheops pyramid and Stonehenge in special places on the earth where invisible yet perceptible energy fields inspire awe and prayer. Power spots and the network of energy lines on the surface of the earth are ascribed to the Metal element.

The trace elements and minerals of the earth are assigned to Metal; without them, growth would be impossible, not to mention the earth's ability to produce nutrients. Earth is the mother; Metal is the father and is responsible for structure, support, and concentration on what is essential. When these two come together, the possibility for birth and growth, in the sense of the element Wood, comes to be.

The Yin organ of Metal is the Lungs; the Yang organ is the Large Intestine. In the Chinese tradition, the Lungs were compared to the first minister of state—the high priest who fulfilled sacred functions which were necessary for the maintenance of order in the community. The Lungs "receive the life energy, the *Qi* of heaven;" the Large Intestine is "the eliminator of waste." In this, the two basic functions of the element Metal can be seen: receiving and releasing the basic forms of energy transfer with our environment.

In the Hindu tradition, the essence of the breath is called the "life energy," or *Prana*, a term that is similar to the Chinese *Qi*. Wilhelm Reich discovered this life energy in his research and called it "Orgone." Modern particle physics uses the term "quantum fields."

Most spiritual traditions use concentration and control of the breath as a meditation technique. In such traditions, the breath is viewed as our connection to the universe, and our conscious use of it as a means to living in harmony with heaven and earth. This is because the breath assumes the middle position between our conscious and unconscious life; the rhythm of the breath is controlled from the center of the autonomic nervous system, yet it can be consciously controlled by any person. Through this, the awareness of the breath is the first, most important step for most people in becoming conscious of the otherwise unconscious processes of the organs.

With every exhalation, the lungs fulfill the most important eliminatory function of the body: the release of carbon dioxide created in the respiratory process. Exhaling means becoming free of toxic substances and creating space for new energy production. One can differentiate between two styles of breathing. One type of person breathes in too much and breathes out too little. They strut around with inflated chests, hold on tightly to what they have, and are often incapable of letting go and relaxing. The other type breathes out more than in. Their chests are collapsed, they suffer from a constant lack of energy, and they constantly look needy, although they have oxygen right in front of their noses.

The double function of the breath—the energetic charge and discharge—is a principle found all over the cosmos. It is the principle of the pulse, the change from expansion to contraction. This principle is found in the behavior of galaxies as well as in the behavior of amoebas and other one-celled organisms. Although concentration is the basic movement of Metal, this does not contradict the principle of pulse or breathing, because it is only by rythmic change from tension to relaxation that a concentration of energy can develop. Rythm is a basic term for Metal. A rhythmic breathing that fully unfolds itself makes the pulse of life in us possible and gives us the power to stay in touch with our environment.

While the Lungs "receive the life energy, the *Qi* of heaven," the Large Intestine is "the eliminator of waste." In this, the two basic functions of the element Metal can be seen: receiving and releasing, the basic forms of energy transfer with our environment.

It is thus clear that the element Metal represents our relationship to the universe—our "connection to heaven." The complementary abilities of receiving and excreting or letting go form the basis of mental and physical health. If the ability to receive is poorly developed, the organism suffers from a deficiency; it is cut off. If the ability to let go is not developed, the organism will become constipated and will stagnate. This is why the Large Intestine is as important as the Lungs for our "connection to heaven"—heaven being a synonym for the mental and spiritual world. Because only if we can let go of mental waste and obsolete mind patterns are we able to grasp fresh ideas and think new thoughts. This is why the functioning of the Large Intestine, on the mental level, means the power of discernment and clarity of thought.

A sign for an imbalance in Metal is an inadequate bond to the environment. People with such an imbalance are often lonely and withdrawn. They seem hard, cold, and isolated from their surroundings, and they show little feeling. Others are ambitious, have high ideals, and strive for something that they can never get. Still others are religious in a fixed and dogmatic way. They have a strong desire to get to heaven. They know many techniques to purify themselves, and they try to convert others to their beliefs and to a pure life. They are, however, incapable of letting themselves go enough to receive the spiritual quality of the essence of Metal. This behavior is understandable when one remembers that the lungs and large intestine make up the most important eliminatory systems in the body, and that, with too little excretion and too shallow breathing, the desire for an inner and outer purification becomes very great. Cleanliness and hygiene fanatics, extreme proponents of macrobiotics, and religious dogmatists are often compensating for their disturbance in Metal with such behavior.

In the fall, the people in simple farm communities are thinking about how they will survive the winter. On gloomy days, they are perhaps worried about the future. An imbalance in Metal is also revealed by a person's exaggerated worry about the future. With a disturbance in Metal, one also finds a pessimistic attitude toward life, a hopelessness. However, if Metal is healthy, then trust in life, optimism, and a positive assessment of the future prevail.

The feeling that corresponds to the fall is sadness. It is the sadness that fills us when we have to take leave of something that has become precious and dear to us. One finds this feeling exaggerated in people who are not able to let go of something that they can never get back. A general sadness can also develop as a result of a weak bond to the world or a lack of vitality and life energy—insufficient *Qi*. We can also feel sad about things that have not yet happened, when we realize that we have not taken advantage of our opportunities.

The tissue that corresponds to Metal is the skin. Here, one can also see the basic principles of this element. The skin is an important eliminatory and breathing organ. We are constantly in touch with our environment through our skin. It responds to the accumulation of waste products by developing various skin diseases and reacting to some environmental stimuli through allergies. We show our attitudes toward other people by allowing them to touch us or by avoiding contact with them. We are in touch with nature only as long as we enjoy the sensation of the coolness of the water and the wind, the warmth of the sun, the softness or roughness of the earth, and the tenderness of the leaves and plants on our skin.

The sensory organ of Metal is the nose. A limited or nonexistent sense of smell points to an imbalance in Metal. The properties of smell are closely connected to the elemental spirit of Metal, called *Po*. With *Po*, the Chinese designate the animal instinct that gives us the ability to smell danger, lets us sense how other people are thinking and feeling about us, and allows us to foresee future events. Our sense of smell makes it possible for us to differentiate between foods, surroundings, and people that may be good or bad for us. It allows us to differentiate between the various scents of flowers and plants. We instinctively reject a person whose smell we do not like, while we feel attracted to a person who smells pleasant, whose fragrance bewitches us.

White is the color assigned to Metal. Most of the time, a white complexion expresses a lack of the Fire element in the personality, a lack of warmth. While Metal is characterized by the striving for intellectual quality, with a deficit in Fire this often turns into a rigid outlook, an intolerant Puritanism, or a religious fanaticism. This type of spirituality lacks enthusiasm, warmth, and spontaneity, characteristics typical of many religions.

It seems to be difficult to live the power of Metal. On the one hand, the core of Metal is concentration, letting go, grief, going within, and leaving the world. On the other hand, it is the connection to our environment, the connection to our vitality, the connection to heaven. Often, we have to withdraw in order to perceive a deeper connection that is not visible in our day-to-day lives. Only when we let go of what was can the circle be completed. Only when we let go, can a space be created in which the old can die and the new can be born. It is important to remove the outer form so that the essence can reveal itself. It is important to let go without giving up, without losing trust. This is how a retreat from the world becomes a retreat into the essential world.

Mental and Physical
Exercises to Refine Metal

CLARIFYING QUESTIONS

Proceed with the questions as you have done previously.

- How do I feel in autumn?
- How do I let go of people or things that have become valuable or dear to me?
- Can I let go of what is gone forever and not surrender myself to false hopes?
- Is it easy for me to withdraw and to concentrate on myself?
- How do I feel when I am alone?
- When was the last time I grieved deeply?
- When was the last time I cried?
- Do I have a sense of what is important in my life?
- Do I have a sense of what is important in my judgment of other people?
- Do others judge me to be a fair person?
- Am I able to clearly formulate sentences and use words skilfully?
- Do I stand on ceremonies and advocate formalities and attention to technicalities?
- Do I insist on ritual politeness?
- Is my behavior sometimes cold and chilly?

- Do I frequently turn down and reject other people?
- Can I smell danger when it is in the air?
- Do I perceive many different smells?
- Do I often have a cold or a flu?
- Do I have a chronic sinus infection?
- Do I tend to strangle feelings by thinking?
- Do I often suffer from bronchitis?
- Have I ever had pneumonia?
- Do I easily get out of breath when I do something strenuous?

METAL EXERCISES

RHYTHM OF THE BREATH AND PERSONALITY Dance to music you like for 15 minutes. Then lie stretched out on your back. Observe the natural rhythm of your breath without influencing it in any way. Establish what type of breather you are: do you exhale more than you inhale (do you have a collapsed, flat chest)? Or do you inhale more, retaining some breath, with more of a rounded, inflated chest? Or is your breathing balanced?

Type I Breather (tendency toward exhalation)
With this kind of breathing, you are likely to run out of energy; you lack stamina. This type of breather is needy, even if the neediness is subtly expressed in the personality. Many times, this neediness is compensated for by special feats and brilliant accomplishments, masked by the consumption of stimulants like nicotine and coffee. Still, this basic feeling forms your life.

A thorough change is attainable only through a change in the rhythm of the breath. The breath forms the basis of your life. The quality of your breath defines the quality of your actions and your experiences, the quality of your thoughts and moods.

Be aware that a thorough change in your breathing rhythm will lead to a drastic and far-reaching transformation of your feelings about life. New possibilities will manifest themselves, perhaps things that you have wished for but couldn't attain. Perspectives you have never thought existed will open themselves to you. But be aware that there might be resistance to doing the following exercises regularly because your organism is accustomed to a certain way of breathing, and all of your mental patterns and emotional habits depend on the way you are breathing now.

The goal of this exercise is to turn your breathing rhythm into its opposite. Breathe in deeply, hold your breath, then breathe out short and shallow, and fill your chest anew with oxygen. Keep repeating this for at least quarter of an hour. For the first few days, it is recommended that you keep the following rhythm: four beats while inhaling, four beats holding your breath, and two beats while exhaling. After this, you can double the sequence: eight beats while inhaling, eight holding your breath, four beats while exhaling.

You can do this exercise while listening to music, driving the car, washing dishes, reading the newspaper, talking, dancing, or playing with children. But if you have trouble doing the exercise for 15 minutes while occupied with other things, then do it in your room where you will not be interrupted.

What is important is the regularity with which you do this. Do the exercise every day for a month and keep a journal about it. Then take stock of what has happened in the meantime. If you have the feeling that it helps you to develop new parts of yourself, do it for three months.

Type II Breather (tendency toward inhalation)

You strut with an inflated chest through the world and like to make a show of your power. You hold on tightly to what you have: your image. It is difficult for you to let go of this image and show your weaknesses. You have learned that you are loved and admired when you are strong. Because of this, you take on a rather stiff and rigid attitude and cannot easily give way or yield. Your life has a somewhat static quality, and perhaps you have wondered why, with all the power you have and all the admiration you receive, you still are not completely satisfied.

If a few of these characteristics are on the mark, try the following exercise: exhale intensely, pause before the next inhalation, take a short and shallow breath, exhale intensely, and so on. For the first few days, follow this rhythm: four beats while exhaling; pause for four beats; two beats while inhaling. Later you can double the rhythm: eight beats while exhaling; pause for eight beats; four beats while inhaling. The rules for the last exercise apply to this one.

APPRECIATING GRIEF   This is a difficult exercise because the ability to grieve and let go is not very well developed in our culture.

At the next opportunity, take time to grieve. It could be at the loss of a relative or a friend, or it could be a bad fight with your partner in which you weren't able to come to an agreement. Withdraw and feel your grief; don't suppress it. In case you don't have a reason to grieve, put yourself in a situation where you become sad: spend some time in an orphanage or a senior care facility.

CONCENTRATING ON WHAT IS IMPORTANT   Write letters to people who mean a lot to you or who have meant a lot to you. Express your feelings and thoughts, above all the conflicts and problems that you have kept to yourself. Try to clear up misunderstandings and concentrate on what is important.

THE LUNG AND LARGE INTESTINE MERIDIANS

STRENGTHENING THE METAL-YIN: THE LUNG POSTURE   This posture embodies the essence of Lung energy: optimism, confidence, and trust in the future.

Take this posture when you feel discouraged and downcast, or when self-doubt blocks you from taking action. While taking this posture, visualize the Lung Meridian. It flows from the shoulder to the thumb. Intensify the energy flow in your imagination with every exhalation.

Activating the Lung Meridian

1. Stand with your feet parallel and three foot-lengths apart, shoulders relaxed, arms hanging down loosely. Your knees should be slightly bent.

2. Stretch your arms out in front of you to the height of your shoulders with your palms facing the ground.

3. While breathing in, swing your arms swiftly as far as possible to the left. Let your hips and your upper body follow. Your head should

follow the movement of your upper body. Imagine that you are hurling something powerfully to the left. Let the motion take you as far as possible behind you in order to attain the greatest extension of the spine and long back muscles. Keep your arms parallel.

4. While breathing out, bring your arms back in front of you to the middle.

5. While breathing in, swing your arms as far as possible to the right (as above), while breathing out, back to the middle.

6. Do this exercise for approximately five minutes.

Mental and Physical Exercises to Refine Metal

STRENGTHENING THE METAL-YANG: THE LARGE INTESTINE POSTURE

This posture speaks for itself. The intellectual function of the large intestine is reflection and the elimination of mental waste: letting go of wishes, expectations, and ideas.

Take this posture when you have the feeling that you have gotten stuck on an idea or when you don't know how to move on.

The energy flows in the Large Intestine Meridian from the index finger, along the outside of the arm and over the shoulder and neck, to a point just next to the nostril. Visualize the flow, white in color, with every inhalation.

Chinese Medicine for Beginners

Activating the Large Intestine Meridian

1. In a standing position, cross your arms over your chest so that the palms of your hands are facing your shoulders.
2. This exercise is called "tightening the bow." While inhaling, straighten and stretch your left arm out to the side (the left hand is holding the bow), and "tighten the string" with your right hand in front of your chest. Your face should be turned to the left, the first finger of your left hand stretched out so that you can see your fingernail. Let the tension build. Through this tension, the Large Intestine Meridian is stimulated.
3. While exhaling, release the arrow from the bow and cross your arms over your chest, as in the beginning of the exercise.
4. Repeat the movements on the right side.
5. Do this exercise for one minute.

Mental and Physical Exercises to Refine Metal

part 6

WATER

The Element Water

THE season of Water is winter, the season of short days and long nights. The land lies under a blanket of snow, and the sun does not warm. Life has withdrawn into the ground; the power of life lies dormant in the seeds. Winter is the period between death and rebirth.

Water was called the "old Yin," the cold darkness. Its feeling is fear—the existential fear associated with survival. Its direction is north, its color black, its time night. The Yin organ of Water is the Kidneys, its Yang organ is the Bladder, and its tissue is the bones.

The character of Water is a sinking below; its energy is a vertical flow to the center of the earth. While the energy of Fire is directed above, toward the sky, Water pulls us into the depths. It acts on the physical body like the force of gravity and leads the soul and life back to its origin, to a deep consciousness, to the central core. The river picks up the stream and leads it back to the sea.

The nature of Water manifests itself in the image of the seed; compressed in a tiny space lies the potential for a large tree, the potential for a divergent development and unfolding. The seed is the essence of the tree. In the Chinese tradition, this essence was designated as the Ancestral Energy. The Kidneys are its guardian. The Ancestral Energy is the quality and quantity of varied energies that one inherits from one's parents and ancestors. The term "Ancestral Energy" is similar to our term "genetic code," whose 64 possible combinations are also found as symbols in the 64 Hexagrams of the *I-Ching*. The kidney is looked upon as the storage space for the Ancestral Energy, and also as a reservoir for different material and fine energies, which, through the intake and processing of food, get into in our organism and cannot be used immediately in life processes. It is said in the *Nei Ching*: "The kidneys receive the essence of *Zang* and *Fu* (organs) and store them."

A few names of points on the Bladder and Kidney Meridians reveal the effect that these points have on the energy storer: Bladder 24, "Conducts the *Qi* to the Sea of Energy"; Bladder 26, "Conducts the Qi to the Sea of Ancestral Energy"; Kidney 1, "Bubbling Spring"; Kidney 6, "Toward the Sea"; Kidney 13, "Nest of Life Force"; and, a point closely associated with the Kidney and Bladder, Governor 4, called *Mingmen*, "Gate of Life."

The traditional Chinese view—that the Kidneys house the genetic constitution—does not contradict the fact that every cell in the organism contains DNA and RNA, because the Kidneys, like any other organ, are seen as a field of force that extends throughout the body. The anatomical kidneys, as well as the bones and the ears, are the places in the body where the "Kidney Energy Field" condenses and materializes. The force of Water, however, like the energy of the other elements, affects every tissue and every cell. On a cellular level, the "Kidney Energy Field" is seen in connection with the chromosomes, the carriers of the genetic constitution. One could say, that the wide variety of structures, forms, and processes found in human, animal, and plant organisms is a result of overlapping and constantly interacting energy fields. In ancient China, the constantly moving fields of forces were called the Elements.

The force of Water is present in various forms in the organism. Water is a flowing building block of the body; it constitutes 65 percent of the body weight and acts as a solvent and a lubricant. In the Chinese tradition, the Kidneys were labeled the controller of the water supply. In farming communities in China, the controller of the water supply held a highly honored position. He regulated the distribution of water for the rice fields in the different municipalities. The constant purification of the organism through water is made possible by the Kidneys, and is one if its most important functions. The flow of water through the body has nothing to do with nourishment; that is the job of the Stomach and Pancreas. Water also doesn't provide the body with life energy, that job is taken care of by the Lungs.

Water flows without color and without form. Throughout the body, it picks up waste products, prevents stagnation, and makes movement, freshness, and "fluidity" of the body possible. There is no bodily function, no life process, that can be carried out without water. The inner secretions require water, and water is needed in the course of the digestive process, wherein food is taken in and transformed into a pulp (this is where the epithet, "Kidneys, Passage to the Stomach," comes from). Water is also needed to moisten the body orifices of eyes, mouth, nose, ears, sexual organs, and anus. And it is necessary for the control of body temperature through perspiration and the maintenance of the joint and muscle fluids.

The taste assigned to Water is salty. Salt regulates the amount of water retained by the body. The salt water of the sea was the place of origin for all life on this planet, and the human body still has an internal sea-water environment, only slightly modified. The physiological mixture of the various salts in the blood and in the tissue fluids is, even after a million years, still similar to the composition of sea water. A surplus of salt in the organism leads to an accumulation of fluid in the tissues and therefore to swelling, edema, and weight gain.

Water rules the bones and, together with the Spleen, the bone marrow. The Kidneys are responsible for maintaining the right composition of salts and minerals in the blood; this is important for the building of the bones as well as for many other life processes. Without the right amount of salts and minerals in the body, the nerves cannot function, the muscles cannot move, and the heart cannot beat. Therefore, it becomes clear why the Chinese find the Kidneys as important as the Heart: The Kidneys ensure the maintenance of the inner environment, the basis of life.

The conduction of nerve impulses especially depends on exact ion concentrations. Because the Kidneys are responsible for maintaining the right balance of ions in the blood and, thus, in the whole body, there is a close connection between the functioning of the Kidneys and the nervous system. This might be why the Chinese assigned the brain and spinal chord to the Water element; in ancient Chinese texts, the brain is called the "Sea of Marrow."

I assume that, two thousand years ago, the Chinese did not know about ion concentrations and neurological processes as we do today. They had a different approach to reality. They thought more in analogies, and their logical processes were more influenced by intuitive insights. Because they did not have the scientific tools that we have today, they had to rely on holistic thinking and insight. Thus, I imagine that the brain was called the "Sea of Marrow," not because of the scientifically provable connection between the functioning of the kidneys and neurological processes, but because the brain in the skull looks very similar to the marrow in the bone. If you have ever observed brain surgery in a movie, you will know what I mean. I assume that they were calling the brain "Sea of Marrow," first, because of a pictorial and also tangible analogy and, second, because they were contemplating the various organs, body tissues, sense organs, and meridians throughout many centuries, and so they had attained an intuitively based and empirically verified knowledge about the connections between the various organs and meridians.

In the context of the nervous system, a few more things can be said about the relationship between Water and Fire. Life evolved in the sea, and the Water element is the base of our life, of our will to survive, of our vitality and sexual drive. The simple life forms are assigned to the Water element: a one-celled organism has no blood circulation and no heart; it is composed of a cell membrane, salt water, genetic material, and simple cell organs. In comparison to this, Fire, along with Metal and Earth, allows a higher order of things to come into being. This is why the material substance of the nervous system is assigned to Water, but the more complex phenomena of the transmission of stimuli and the coordination of electrical impulses in the nervous system are attributed to Fire. Water is the base, Fire is the top.

In the Chinese tradition, all of the hormones and glands are associated with the Water element. The ancient texts distinguish Yin-Kidney and Yang-Kidney. The Yin-Kidney is also called the Water-Kidney, and the Yang-Kidney the Fire-Kidney.

The Water-Kidney filters the blood and produces urine. On the physical level, it corresponds to the kidney with all its various functions as we know it in Western medicine. The Fire-Kidney corresponds to the endocrine system: the adrenal glands, the sex glands, the islets of Langerhans in the pancreas, the thyroid and thymus, and, finally, the pituitary gland.

The concept of the Water-Kidney and Fire-Kidney also indicates the nature of the elemental spirit of Water, the *Zhen*. *Zhen* is our will power, our will to survive, and our sexual drive. It represents the vitality with which a person masters life. *Zhen* can unfold when the organism is flowing freely, fresh and clean inside, and when the hormones are working so well together that the metabolic processes are well tuned. Then a bubbly, fiery power and vitality can develop. This power manifests itself in supple body movements, flexible joints, sexual potency, strong bones and healthy teeth, a silky shine to the hair, good hearing, a tremendous urge for action and activity, and a healthy ability to adjust to the demands of circumstances. The balance of the element Water is dependent upon the relationship between the Yin-Kidney and the Yang-Kidney. When the Yang-Kidney is weak, or when there is surplus energy in the Yin-Kidney in contrast to the Yang-Kidney, the will to live, vitality, and sexual drive decrease. The results may be a general weakness, impotence, frigidity, and paralyzing fear.

When the energy of the Yang-Kidney is dominant, one often finds a person who is constantly in a hurry or a person with rigid behavior and body movements. This rigidity and stiffness manifests itself, above all, in the lower back, the ilio-sacral joints, and the backs of the legs along the course of the Bladder Meridian. The symptoms of this rigidity are a hollow back, disk problems in the lumbar vertebrae, sciatica, lumbago, and bladder infections.

Other consequences of an imbalance in Water are kidney stones, kidney and urinary tract infections, bone diseases, loss of hair, some types of watery diarrhea, menstrual disorders, insomnia, and constantly cold legs and feet.

The Kidneys rule the ears and hearing. The balance of the fluid in the ear is crucial to the quality of our hearing. Our sense of balance—a function made possible by the right combination of fluid in the labyrinth of the ear—is also assigned to Water. Most illnesses concerning the ears—inflammation of the middle ear, buzzing in the ears, hearing difficulties, deafness, or dizziness—can be traced to a disturbance in the Water element.

The hormones produced by the adrenal glands and their function explains the emotions and drives associated with Water. On the one hand, there are the androgens with their direct effect on the libido; on the other hand, there are adrenaline, noradrenaline, cortisol, and aldosterone, which regulate blood pressure and the balance of fluids in the body. A real or imagined danger that causes us to be afraid is the strongest stimulus that sets off the release of these hormones in the circulatory system. In China, fear is associated with the tremendous power of Water, which shows itself in floods set off by earthquakes and tidal waves triggered by typhoons. Fear is also associated with a Water deficiency, such as when the fields dry out and famine is imminent.

As with the other elements, there are emotions and feelings associated with the force of Water that express a balance or imbalance in this element. When one has all five senses together and balanced, it is natural to feel afraid in dangerous situations. We are afraid of something concrete; we recognize the danger in time and can take action to get away from what is threatening us. Fear ensures our biological survival. Through fear we learn to respect life and its awesome power.

Compared to fear, anxiety and terror are more intense; they are emotional states in which the actual threat can no longer be properly assessed. Often, the threat is imaginary and illusory. Anxiety is a state in which either a threat cannot be judged correctly, or the danger no longer exists. The word "anxiety" stems from the Latin word *angustia*, which can be translated as "narrowness, restriction, conciseness, difficulty, poverty, need, and trouble." Anxieties develop when we have isolated ourselves and are no longer in harmony with things and people around us. Being able to resonate with our environment is a characteristic of the Water element: to be soft, to surrender oneself, and to not put up any resistance. Serious disturbances in Water lead to panic attacks, paranoia, a persecution complex, fear of the dark, fear of an inner "black hole," and situations in which one becomes rigid, immovable, and paralyzed with fear.

The Water element harbors the deepest secrets of life. When we accept the power of Water, we become quiet inside and the surface of the lake becomes smooth. In this inner quiet, the world of dreams, the realms of sleep, and the unconscious slowly open up. Step by step, the way through the realm of death also becomes visible. Water is the element of the deepening of self and meditation. If one is at home in the depths, one can meet the storms on the surface calmly. With Water, more than with any other element, we come across that which has no name, the *Tao*.

Mental and Physical
Exercises to Get the
Water Flowing

CLARIFYING QUESTIONS

Proceed with the following questions as you have done previously.

- How do I feel in winter or when the weather is cold?
- Do I have a fear of the dark?
- Do I have a strong will that helps me to overcome difficulties?
- Do I have a strong or a weak sex drive?
- In what situations do I deeply relax?
- Can I delve into something to a point where everything else loses its meaning?
- Do I have a strong imagination or ability to fantasize?
- What am I afraid of?
- Do I have secrets?
- Do I hear well?
- Have I ever had inflammation of the middle ear or a buzzing in the ears that lasted for a long time?
- Is my hair healthy and strong?
- Are my teeth good?

- Do I sometimes have discomfort or pain in the small of my back?
- Do I tend to get bladder infections?
- Have I ever had an illness of the kidneys?
- Do I prefer salty food, or do I have an aversion to salt?
- Am I very ambitious, or not ambitious at all?
- What or whom do I respect or revere?
- What really amazed me last week?
- Have I ever thought about how I will die or how I would like to die?
- What is my attitude toward death?
- What do I think is the biggest secret in life?

WATER EXERCISES

CONFRONTING YOUR FEAR   Go into a dark room in the evening. Imagine a situation in which you were afraid, and call it back into your memory in detail. Let the situation appear worse to you than it was, and enter into your fear.

When you feel the fear deeply, focus your attention on your body. Where do you get cramped and tense? Do you hold your breath or take short, shallow breaths? Take a few deep, long breaths while you once again experience the fearful situation in your imagination. Keep breathing deeply until the fear lessens or completely disappears.

If you are a fearful person, do this exercise once a week for one to two months. It can help reduce your fears. Then, next time a dangerous situation arises, you will be able to react more calmly and defend yourself better.

FEELING THE WOMB   Lie down on your bed in the afternoon or evening and close your eyes. Take approximately 15 minutes to journey into your past. Remember how you felt yesterday, a week ago, a year ago, three years ago, five years ago, and so on. Remember your puberty, your first years of school, your childhood. Imagine how you might have felt as an infant, at your birth, before your birth. If feelings or pictures from this time appear, let them come; do not try to interpret them or compare them to what you already know. Imagine that you are swimming in amniotic fluid. Then feel the slow, deep breaths of your mother as she sleeps, and how they rock you tenderly. Imagine this breath that surrounds you and is bigger than you, that rocks you and keeps you safe. And then let your own tiny breath become synchronized with this bigger breath. Simply listen to it; don't do anything else. The breath goes in. The breath goes out. The breath goes in. The breath goes out.

Listen for about 15 minutes to the breath in the silence.

LATIHAN This is a technique of the *Tantra* tradition. It releases the "flow of water" in us—the ability to be soft, to be yielding, to let things happen, to flow.

Go into a dark room in the evening. Wear comfortable clothes and take off your shoes and socks. Dance a fantasy dance for 15 minutes so that you become loose and relaxed.

Then stand in the middle of the room and don't move; don't do anything. Remain loose, but refrain from moving. After a few minutes, you will sense that your body begins to stir on its own. Let it move exactly as it wants to; don't interfere. Perhaps you will feel a twitch, or a small quiver may go through your body. A movement begins, is interrupted, and then continues. Follow the dynamic of your body.

After a while, you will feel charged. Whenever you turn off your arbitrary motor, deeper centers in the brain take over the controls, and suppressed movements can come to the surface. Tension and blocks eventually release themselves under the influence of self-regulated centers, and the muscle tone changes. Energy is released.

Remain in this state for about 30 minutes. Then lie on your back and enjoy the relaxed feeling you have.

THE BLADDER AND KIDNEY MERIDIANS

STRENGTHENING THE WATER-YANG: THE BLADDER POSTURE The function of the Bladder has to do with mental and physical relaxation, letting go of activity, and returning to a quiet state.

Take this posture when you have done strenuous work and would like to relax. Swing slowly from one side to the other and back again.

Then change the direction for a while. Let your upper body fall effortlessly forward, then stand up again and arch backward to stretch your back and neck muscles. Do this several times.

With every repetition, let your body fall farther forward while visualizing the Bladder Meridian. It flows from the inner corner of the eye, over the head, down the back and the backs of the legs, along the outside of the foot to the small toe. Visualize it on your head and your back approximately two finger-widths to either side of the midline of your body.

Activating the Bladder Meridian: The Candle and the Plow
1. The candle: Lie relaxed on your back, your arms at your sides.
2. Raise your legs to a vertical position.
3. Supporting your back with your hands, lift your lower torso so that it lies on the same vertical line as the legs. The weight of your body rests on your shoulders and neck. Each day, stay a bit longer in this posture, up to three minutes.

Mental and Physical Exercises to Get the Water Flowing

4. Then proceed slowly to the plow: keeping your legs straight, slowly bring them over your head until your toes are touching the ground. Hold your legs as straight as you can without feeling a painful tension. Relax and breathe into your abdomen. Remain in this position for up to three minutes.

5. Keeping your legs straight, raise them slowly back to a vertical position until you are in the candle posture again.

6. Lower your legs slowly until you are lying on your back. Take at least a minute to relax and enjoy the effects of this exercise. The candle and the plow are Hatha Yoga exercises that stretch and activate the Bladder Meridian. They loosen the spine, the cramped muscles in the neck and back, and the backs of the legs. They relieve the heart by promoting blood flow in the veins and preventing edema in the legs and varicose veins.

Chinese Medicine for Beginners

STRENGTHENING THE WATER-YIN: THE KIDNEY POSTURE This position depicts the essence of the Kidneys: trust, flow, regeneration, and quiescence.

The Kidney Meridian flows from the sole of the foot along the inside of the leg to the pelvic floor, and from there it ascends along the spine to the lower back. From *Mingmen* (Governor 4), at the level of the second lumbar vertebra, it goes to the kidneys and, along the ureters, to the bladder. It comes to the surface of the body again at the upper border of the pubic bone and ascends from there along the abdomen and the chest up to the collar bone. Visualize the Kidney Meridian in the bent leg while you breathe in (the energy flow is less intense in the straight leg).

Take the mirror-image of this posture for a while and visualize the Kidney Meridian on the other side.

Mental and Physical Exercises to Get the Water Flowing

Activating the Kidney Meridian

1. Sit on the floor with your legs bent, so that the soles of your feet are touching each other.
2. Hold your ankles and press the Kidney 6 point with your thumbs on both feet. This acupressure point lies one thumb-width under the tip of the inner ankle bone in the small indentation between the tendons.
3. Pull your feet as close to your pelvis as possible.
4. When you inhale, sit up and stretch your spine. When you exhale, bend your upper body, bringing your forehead as close to your toes as possible.
5. Do this exercise for a minute. Breathe deeply and regularly.
6. When you are finished, sit up straight with your legs crossed and close your eyes. When you exhale, say the mantra "Zhen" to yourself for one to three minutes.

Chinese Medicine for Beginners

part 7

THE FOUR CYCLES

THE Chinese placed a great deal of importance on the harmony and balance of the forces and energies. For the observed processes in nature and the cosmos, the characteristics of the individual elements play less of a role than their actual interplay. In every life process, the elements balance each other, create each other, and block each other. The Chinese tradition recognizes four laws governing the relationship of the elements to each other: The Cycle of Creation (*Sheng*), The Cycle of Checking-Up and Control (*Ko*), The Cycle of Rebellion, and The Cycle of Withdrawal.

These four cycles describe the phases of growth and the physiological interplay of the organs. They describe the path and the spreading of complaints and diseases from one element to another, from one organ to another. The four cycles make the complex combinations that form the basis for the individual clinical pictures understandable. If one applies them to the emotional and mental levels, one gets an overview of the dialectic between feelings and mental attitudes.

The cycles also describe the personality structures as well as the connection between personality and illness. They are a basic instrument of traditional Chinese diagnosis and therapy. The four cycles show how the elements are connected to each other, and how everything that happens has an effect on everything else.

THE *SHENG* CYCLE OR
THE LAW OF MOTHER AND CHILD

This cycle describes the transition from one element to the next, from one phase to the next. Wood transforms into Fire, Fire into Earth, Earth into Metal, Metal into Water, and Water back into Wood. In Chinese texts, the changes are shown in the following way: you use wood to make fire; when the fire has burned, it becomes ashes, it becomes earth; in the depths of the earth, metals and minerals are compressed and created; water condenses on metal, or out of heaven, the kingdom of metal, comes the rain; water nourishes the plants so they can grow, hence, water creates wood; when a lot of wood is piled up, then the fire will burn brighter and longer; the burning of fields creates new, fertile earth. The manifestation of energy of every element is dependent upon the nourishment it gets from the element before it in the cycle; therefore, this cycle is also called The Cycle of Nourishment.

Nourishment and building are attributed to the Yin, so the *Sheng* cycle is particularly effective in the Yin organs. The Liver (Wood Yin) nourishes the Heart, the Heart (Fire Yin) nourishes the Spleen, the Spleen (Earth Yin) nourishes the Lungs, the Lungs (Metal Yin) nourish the Kidneys, the Kidneys (Water Yin) nourish the Liver, and so on.

It is difficult to translate the principles described here into terms understood in Western physiology. The *Sheng* cycle describes the transformation of dynamic powers and energies that have reflections on the organic and mental levels. It is not possible to measure the energies, but one can recognize their effects.

For example, in the practice of Chinese medicine, the Kidneys are strengthened through the Lung energy. This combination is often found in illnesses. If the first imbalances and illnesses in childhood are in Metal and are manifested in chronic colds, whooping cough, pneumonia or diarrhea, then, in the next period of growth, one is likely to find imbalances in Water, manifested in middle-ear infections, buzzing in the ears, or tooth decay. In this case, Water and its organs and tissues were undernourished for years because Metal was weak.

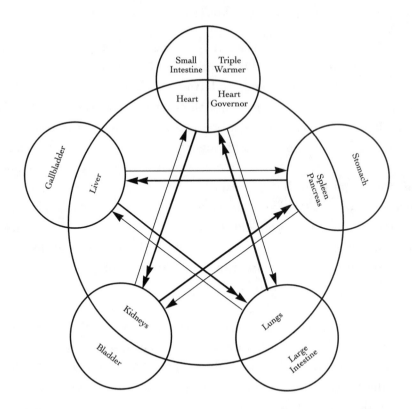

The *Sheng* cycle portrays a closed circle. If the circle is broken at any point and one element is unable to nourish the next, the result is "malnourishment." The Chinese call this, relative to the previous element, the "child." The nourishing element is the "mother." The child of one element is the mother of the next, and so on, until the circle is completed. Therefore, this cycle is called The Law of Mother and Child. The strength of an element is dependent on proper nourishment from the mother. One can observe this mother-child relationship in every area—biological, emotional, and mental. Undernourishment is important for diagnosis, but there are also diseases caused by overfeeding.

As clear as these laws may appear in an individual case, it is difficult to describe them abstractly. On an emotional level, one can best understand the transition of the feelings from one element to the next when one looks at the course of the year with its different seasons and the basic feelings that are associated with them. Spring is the time for new plans; new projects are started. People are more extroverted; they meet new people and fall in love anew. As the whole emotional spectrum of Wood is intensified during spring, some people may experience increased impatience and irritability on one hand if the Wood element is strong, and deep depression on the other hand if the Wood element is weak. The blooming of summer grows out of this new beginning in spring—the joy of succeeding, celebrating, and dancing. A person may feel relieved and conciliatory after a sudden release of anger; one has expressed oneself, stated one's opinion, and not stood in one's own way. The experience shows that people who never become angry rarely experience a real, pulsating joy. One can readily observe the transition from Wood to Fire in children. One minute they are hopping mad, insulting each other, arguing or fighting with each other, and the next minute they are best friends again and play as if there had never been anything wrong.

After a time of joy, we often linger in its wake and yearn to return to it. We become quieter, more reflective, maybe even melancholic. We rave about romance and experiences from the past. These are all moods of the element Earth. Empathy and sympathy can arise out of fully felt joy—a deep understanding and bonding with someone you love and with whom you have shared happiness. Out of the sympathy that has arisen from a shared high or peak experience, constructive criticism becomes possible—yet another characteristic of the element Earth.

Melancholy can result in sadness; empathy can lead to insight about whether and when it would be a good time to leave another person. A person who can feel the needs of another will know when it is time to go. Such a person will also know the right time to be alone and to draw within, not clinging to the other person, as is common with a person who has an overly strong Earth with a disturbed transition into Metal. A person who experiences a flowing transition from Earth to Metal is able to let go of the past, sever past bonds, and give up old identities. The essence of past experiences will be kept, and those that are not important will be released. Maturity will develop through grieving and letting go. If the transition from Metal to Water is incomplete, then the person will be afraid of being alone. Aloneness will be seen as loneliness and a yearning to bond with others. Behind the fear of loneliness is almost always the fear of being confronted with oneself and one's own unconscious. This is so because, in being alone, we experience through our own power who we really are. The ability assigned to the Metal element of letting go and taking leave of something or someone is necessary in order to arrive at the stillness of the Water and to become silent.

Out of the silence grows a new beginning. This is the transition from Water to Wood. On an emotional level, we experience this transition as a sudden change from fear to aggression. A person who is cornered and feels threatened may, out of fear, suddenly attack or feel paralyzed. The former shows a healthy transition from Water to Wood. One can see this especially clearly in animals and children. With inhibited people who were raised to be well-behaved and to hold themselves back, the paralyzing form of fear dominates. One cannot imagine a way out or how to successfully prevail. The transition from Water to Wood is unbalanced. Plants cannot grow from salt water.

THE *KO* CYCLE OR THE
LAW OF GRANDMOTHER AND GRANDCHILD

The cycle of creation and building has, as its natural polarity, breakdown and destruction of outlived structures. Everything that grows has its natural limits beyond which the growth is no longer useful. If these limits are exceeded, an imbalance in the elements results, causing rampant growth, hypertrophy, and finally cancer.

Just as every element has a mother who nourishes it, every element also has a grandmother who is responsible for its upbringing and its proper growth. In ancient China, as in many other cultures, the grandparents had the job of recognizing the proper vocation for their grandchildren and furthering this by taking care of the training. They were the real authorities in the upbringing; they passed on the experience of generations, mostly in the form of narration or stories. They made the decisions concerning career and marriage. The parents, in contrast, took care of the material side of life; they worked in the fields and supported the family.

It is characteristic of our culture that the function of the grandparents, especially in cities, has become almost meaningless. The education and development of children is put in the hands of anonymous public schools, where a lot of information is given, but very little real knowledge is conveyed about one's destiny and the meaning of life. What remains is the function of the parents, who take care of supporting the family materially.

It was the job of the grandparents to give their grandchildren the direction and support necessary for their development. If the grandparents were too strict and their methods too authoritarian, the grandchildren did not develop independence in actions, thoughts, and feelings. If they let their grandchildren get away with too much and did not reprimand them enough, the grandchildren became too high-handed, arrogant, and incapable of being subordinate later in life.

The diagram of the *Ko* cycle shows a five-pointed star. In the mystical traditions of the Western world, this symbol is known as a pentagram—the symbol of white magic when it is right-side up, and the symbol of black magic when it is upside down. Like the *Sheng* cycle, the *Ko* cycle, The Cycle of Control, is a system of abstract symbols that makes it possible to connect empirical observations and ideas from very different areas with one another. In the Chinese texts, the laws of the *Ko* cycle were portrayed in the following manner: water puts out fire, fire melts metal, metal (in the form of a saw or ax) cuts wood, wood (as a plant or tree) breaks through the surface of the earth, earth dams up the path of water.

Too much water extinguishes the fire completely. One finds this relationship between Water and Fire in people who are ambitious, driven, and strong-willed, but who lack warmth, joy, and a bright quality. This can also be seen in people who are full of fear and paranoia; fear is the opponent of love.

Too little water allows the fire to blaze too high. The fire consumes itself too quickly and results in a flash in the pan instead of a warming fire. The consequences on the emotional level are overenthusiasm, mania

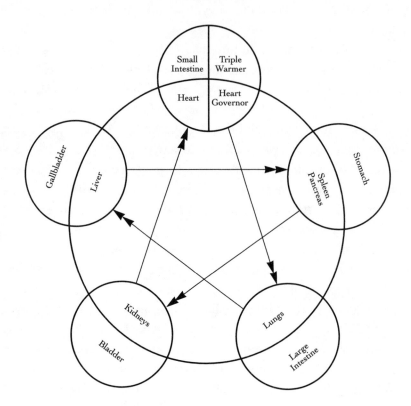

and hysteria, and carousing and revelry, which turn to depression after the fire has burned out. Other signs of this sort of imbalance are insomnia and unstable moods.

Fire melts metal. Fire is necessary in order to give metal a form, in order to refine it. Practical tools and jewelry can be created. The elasticity and hardness of many metals are dependent upon their temperature; in extreme cold they become brittle, while in warmer temperatures they are more flexible and resistant. To the mental qualities of Metal, to the striving for purity and spirituality, the warmth of Fire adds enthusiasm, serenity, cheerfulness, and joy that are characteristic of a truly religious person. Too little Fire leads to zealotry. Too much Fire leads to religious hysteria and rapture, to vagueness and obscurity of the mind; the feeling for what is essential in life is lost. On an emotional level, Fire might be able to cheer up a sad person and get them to smile. A joke often helps one get over low spirits and dejectedness.

Metal cuts wood. The polarity of expansion and contraction, of spring and fall, characterizes this relationship. People with an overly strong Metal give the impression of being withdrawn or cut off and isolated from their surroundings. It often appears as if they are carrying around sadness from their childhood, expressed in their pale complexion. They have a tendency to let their shoulders droop. They are marked by a fearfulness and a pessimistic attitude that block them from making a fresh start and being courageous. It is difficult for them to dedicate themselves to new projects and to meet new people. They don't take the necessary risks to get what they want, and they don't allow themselves to be aggressive. They would rather have their sad face than a purifying thunderstorm, and sometimes rationalize this through a religious doctrine.

In contrast, too little Metal allows the Wood to grow wild. This type of person lives expansively and takes on new adventures again and again. Such a person will be full of entrepreneurial spirit and inventiveness, but will sometimes become lost in the activities; a sense of what is really important might be lacking at times.

Wood penetrates the earth. If the forest or jungle covers an entire country, then there is hardly any room for fertile fields. If there is no forest, the soil will not be able to hold moisture, the minerals will be washed away, and the country will be transformed into a desert or steppe. Wood is the grandmother of the earth; it is responsible for its fertility. The relationship between Wood and Earth is characterized by the polarity of activity and receptivity. If a person is too active, making too many plans, taking on too many projects, and having too many decisions to make, then many of these projects will not be able to mature, and it will be difficult to find peace within. People who are not rooted may travel a lot or feel as if they are always on the go. This way of life can lead to irritability and insecurity. The Earth element provides a feeling of security. Wood that is too strong brings with it an overall aggressiveness; where there is a lot of aggression, there is little room for empathy and sympathy, little readiness to care for others and to be there for them.

In contrast, if Wood is weak and cannot control the Earth, then a *Shi* state of the spleen results: an overprotectiveness of others, an effusive romanticism, or a constant brooding over what one failed to do in life because one did not assert oneself, carry through, and succeed.

Earth cuts off the path of water. The picture of this relationship is a dam that regulates the flow of water. It prevents the water from flooding the land after a heavy rainfall. The interplay between earth and water ensures that there is enough water for the fields for the whole year. On a human level, this expresses itself as the polarity of having both a sense of reality and deep, uncontrollable feelings—the polarity of practicality and reason, mysticism and sensitivity. On the one hand, there is the Earth with its sense of what is important in life, and on the other hand, the element Water with its tendency toward dreams, music, drugs, deep feelings, and sinking into the unconscious.

A person in whom the Earth element is too strong will have priorities such as: keeping the house in order, fulfilling job responsibilities correctly, earning money, and getting recognition. This recognition will be obtained by observing the morals and ethics of the culture, not necessarily because of an inherent feeling of right and wrong or personal values. This focus on material things doesn't leave much room for arriving at a deeper understanding of the Water element, which will be repressed, perhaps through fighting. This type of person often makes sweeping judgments about meditation, hypnosis, drugs, and ecstatic feelings. Fear of one's own suppressed feelings is usually the basis for this kind of behavior.

If the Earth element is too weak and can no longer regulate the flow of Water, it results in a flood of the psyche—a flood of feelings over which one has no control. One gets flooded by strong feelings and becomes afraid of having the rug pulled out from under one's feet. Deep feelings are often accompanied by this fear of losing control over one's life and one's actions. This fear goes away only when one has learned to trust Water and destiny.

If the element Water predominates, it results in a feeling of being at the mercy of society and of not being able to control one's own emotions. Inner turbulence and unreasonable fears can become as strong as a tidal wave. These existential fears are a constituting element in drug addiction, schizophrenia, and psychosis.

The *Ko* cycle also determines the relationship between Yang and Yin in the organism. The "grandmother" Yang organ controls the "grandchild" Yin organ. For example, the Gall Bladder controls the Spleen, the Stomach controls the Kidneys, and so on. Hyperfunction and hypofunction of the Gall Bladder will adversely affect the energy system of the Spleen-Pancreas and, in many cases, damage it. Simply stated, one could say that hyperfunction of the Gall Bladder energy leads to a suppression of the energy cycle in the Spleen. With hypofunction, the energy system of the Spleen becomes too strong and thus will also become imbalanced.

The *Ko* cycle ensures that a balance of energy among the elements can be reached and maintained, in nature and in humans. Through this cycle, the growth of each individual element is limited to such an extent that organic, useful growth can come about.

If one applies the *Ko* cycle to the emotional level, it becomes clear that the basic human feelings are all equally important—not only for emotional balance, but also for the balance and stability of the physical body and the spiritual self—as these three levels are in constant interaction. Annoyance, anger, laughter, joy, sympathy, melancholy, sadness, grief, lust, and fear all are of the same value in our life, because they are constitutional energies of ourselves and are the expression of the five elemental forces that create and form our body, mind, and soul. A person whose elements are balanced will be able to feel and follow all of these emotional impulses.

It is obvious that, in our culture, joy and compassion are well received most of the time, while anger, lust, grief, and fear are not. This attitude has far-reaching consequences, as all of the basic emotions that are judged negatively, suppressed, or repressed by an individual or society will, according to the laws of the *Sheng* and *Ko* cycles, severely disturb the delicate interplay of the elements. People who never show annoyance and anger may be pleasant to others, but this behavior affects not only their element Wood, but also directly affects their Fire and Earth. They will probably show little warmth and spontaneity, and will feel very little true joy in life. They try to be pleasant and obliging toward others, but their bodies will express this imbalance. They may tend toward obesity, diabetes, gastritis, or other diseases of the Earth element.

Many analogous examples could be listed. A person who cannot laugh and cry, a person who cannot be furious and fearful, a person who cannot sense the worries of others is missing a power and cannot live life fully. Every one-sided predominance of certain feelings—certain ways of thinking and behavioral patterns—results in an imbalance of the elements. This increases with time and undermines one's well-being, later leading to uneasiness and unhappiness and eventually, when the imbalance is no longer experienced consciously, to chronic physical illnesses. The majority of the diseases of civilization (migraines, back problems, menstrual disorders, high blood pressure, heart attacks, diabetes, and so forth) arise in this way. They develop in a process that takes years or decades. They mirror the uneasiness within this culture, the burden of civilization.

THE CYCLE OF REBELLION

The cycle of rebellion is described in the Chinese tradition as the "grandchild who rebels against the grandmother."

If too much energy is in Wood, then Wood first damages Earth (through the *Ko* cycle). However, an overly strong Wood could also rebel against Metal and bring this element out of balance. That is the relationship of the strong, impudent grandchild to its grandmother; the grandchild has lost respect for the grandmother and therefore confronts her methods of upbringing.

A surplus of Wood can create an illness in the Earth element as well as an illness or disturbance in Metal. This is how a person whose attention is basically directed toward work and career, who constantly has to prevail, maintain a position of power, and make precise decisions, will display an imbalance in Metal. In later years, such a person may be incapable of giving up the identity of the successful entrepreneur, breaking down and dying soon after retirement, or being incapable of grief or tears.

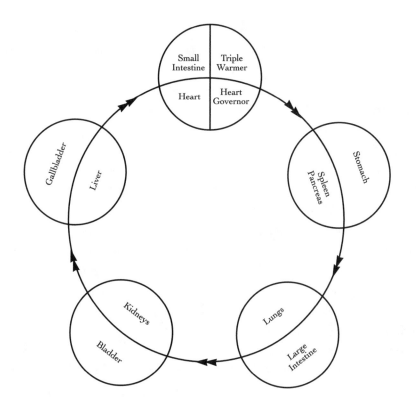

The Cycle of Withdrawal

This law is rather graphically described as the "child who damages the mother" or as the "greedy child who sucks the mother dry."

If the energy of an element has been constantly used up by a bad habit, by unbalanced character traits, or by particular stress on this element because of chronic illness, then too much energy can be withdrawn from the nourishing mother-element via the *Sheng* cycle. Then, the mother herself becomes weak and sick. To give an example: through a sedentary life, constant reading, brooding, thinking, or a chronic Earth-element illness, not only is the Earth weakened, but also Fire, because the Earth, using up more energy than is available within the Earth element, takes the missing energy from the mother—as long as it is there. The child sucks the mother dry. This can, under certain circumstances, also lead to an illness of the Fire element. The mother who spends half her life taking care of her family, who constantly has to sympathize with everyone, will eventually lose her *joie de vivre* if she does not have a strong personality and inner resources. Another example would be the civil servant or bookkeeper who loses more zest for life with every year spent doing the same thing.

The following example clarifies the role that the four cycles can play in the emergence of an illness. In many cases, a lung disease will be directly due to an emotional or physiological imbalance in Metal. However, the same lung disease can also arise from an imbalance in the Spleen ("the mother does not give the child enough nourishment"). It can come about through sick Kidneys ("the child withdraws energy from the mother"). Also, an imbalance in the Fire element—a heart defect or arteriosclerosis—can cause the lung disease ("the grandmother is too soft or too hard on the grandchild"). Eventually, it can arise from an imbalance in Wood ("the grandchild rebels against the grandmother").

With this example, one can see how important an exact diagnosis of the cause of a disease is, as this diagnosis determines the starting point of therapy. Hence, chronic bronchitis will sometimes be treated through Earth, in another case through Fire, and in yet another case through the Lungs and Large Intestine, the Metal organs.

The element from which the illness or imbalance arises can be detected through the fine methods of diagnostics that are a part of Chinese medicine. Diagnosis is beyond the scope of this book, but suffice it to say that chronic symptoms can only be healed when one has found the original cause of the disorder and treated it.

Serious and acute symptoms, such as high fever, circulatory collapse, or intense pain, almost always require a direct, "symptomatic" treatment first, especially when the situation is life-threatening. Only afterward can a doctor attend to the cause of the disorder.

The success of traditional Chinese medicine in treating chronic illnesses is, for the most part, based on restoring the balance of the elements. In many cases, this is possible via knowledge of the four cycles and help from suitable therapeutic methods: diet, herbal extracts, breathing and physical exercises, meridian massage, *Shiatsu,* acupressure, acupuncture, and meditation.

PRACTICAL USE OF THE CYCLES

This section on the four cycles can help you to make the right decision when choosing the exercises that best correspond to your needs. You will also be able to understand and interpret events and experiences in your life when you perform the exercises regularly.

The sequence of the exercises is also important. It is advantageous to arrange the exercises according to the *Sheng* cycle, beginning with Wood and ending with Water. This is relevant if you do all or most of the exercises—the emotional and mental as well as the physical exercises. If you decide to explore the nature of the Five Elements, start by doing the exercises for the element that seems to be weakest in your personality. If it is not obvious with which element to start, start with Wood. Focus on each element, in the order of the *Sheng* cycle, for some time—maybe for a week or two—to really experience the individual quality and power of each element.

In merely doing the physical exercises that stimulate energy flow through the organs and their meridians, it is recommended that you proceed in the order of the *Qi* flow through the meridians. The circulation of *Qi* in the twelve organ meridians has its own sequence. It is different from the laws of the four cycles described in this chapter. *Qi* flows in the meridians in the following order: from Lung to Large Intestine to Stomach to Spleen to Heart to Small Intestine to Bladder to Kidney to Pericardium to Triple Warmer to Gall Bladder to Liver —and from the Liver Meridian, the circulating *Qi* flows back to the Lung Meridian to start a new cycle. The circulation of *Qi* in the body is a continuous flow similar to the blood circulation.

If you want to enhance your energy to get going for the day, to feel healthy and alive, do the physical exercises to stimulate the *Qi* flow in the meridians. As in working with the elements, select the meridian exercises of those organs that seem to be weaker than others. Select between six and twelve exercises, and pause after each posture for a moment with your eyes closed to feel the specific effect.

Afterword

Every time period and every culture has its Achilles heel. The Achilles heel of the twentieth century is the continual poisoning of our planet and its atmosphere and the ever-growing threat posed to nature by humans who, through our search for prosperity and material security, are destroying the basic support systems needed for our lives and those of the plants and other animals. Technology and civilized living, created to protect us from natural catastrophes, have gotten the upper hand to the extent that things are out of balance. We are now left with the question of how we can protect ourselves from technology and civilization.

In the eighteenth and nineteenth centuries, class differences and contrasts in the standard of living were a source of tension in social structures in Europe and the United States. These disparities led to enormous changes and revolutions, from the French Revolution to the growth of communism in Eastern Europe. In the second half of the twentieth century, ecological problems have pushed their way to the forefront. In these times, in Europe and North America, the confrontation between humans and nature has become as important as the confrontations among human beings, if not more so.

The earth is a living being—an enormous organism, say the Hopi Indians. In the twentieth century it is sick, and the nature spirits have withdrawn into the earth. It is possible that the earth will cramp up and shake itself loose until she can once again breathe freely.

Humanity can be seen as the brain of the earth, the carrier of a certain form of intelligence and rationality; humans are the gray and white ganglion cells of the earth organism. The ganglion cells are capable of learning very quickly from each other and passing on their experiences to other parts of the nervous system. They are capable of imagining changes and manifesting them, thereby influencing and changing other parts of the organism.

It is similar in the human organism. Humans are capable of following their intellect, even when it is not in the best interest of the body. A child can be so fascinated by the discovery of the world of its mind that it forgets everything else around it. The more it reads and thinks, the more it will feel at home in the world of ideas. Eventually, it will consider its thoughts to be reality; the ideas it has about life become life itself. At some point, it will take it one step farther and no longer trust its own senses if these speak against the concept it has built up in its mind.

One can compare how most people in Western cultures treat their bodies with how most of humanity treats the earth. Many people in the West no longer know how it feels to be *in* their bodies, to be a body. They do not know what it is like to perceive the world directly with their senses. They *have* a body, but they are not this body. They confuse thinking about life with life itself.

Just as Western medicine is helpless in the face of many chronic diseases of civilization, we also feel helpless in regard to making decisions about our dying forests and other environmental disasters. Our society is just as powerless in trying to stop cancer, AIDS, arteriosclerosis, diabetes, arthritis, allergies, and skin diseases as it is in trying to stop the destruction of rivers, forests, and the soil through chemical products, heavy metals, and radioactivity. We have not yet come to our senses, or we would have revolted a long time ago.

What should we do? Where should we begin? How can we turn back the clock to a time when people were not separate from nature, to a time when there was no split between body and soul?

There are only a few people in the world today who are aware of the dimensions of these problems. At best, one can expect a form of plastic surgery from the leaders in government, industry, and education, and unfortunately no real change in thought or behavior. Only an ecological catastrophe would force them to quickly and thoroughly change their way of thinking and replace the mostly material goals of our prosperity-minded society with goals that are more in tune with life on this planet.

What to do? What position do we have to take to help save the planet? What things do we have to refrain from doing? Can we wait for our politicians and environmental conferences to make decisions? It seems that the political system that could pass effective laws to reduce the emissions of carbon dioxide, to reduce the poisoning of the rivers and the sea, to save the ozone layer, and so forth, is in the grip of the various economic lobbies. The measures taken so far against global pollution and the disintegration of the Earth's biological systems are totally inadequate and incomplete. Can we afford to wait for our politicians to do the enormous job of passing hundreds of environmental laws that would go totally against the ways and the ideals of the affluent society? It seems that our politicians are unable to do it. One of the reasons might be that they only are the tip of the iceberg —the iceberg being the Judeo-Christian culture stream that turned against nature three thousand years ago, declaring that humanity should be separate from the plant and animal kingdoms and that Earth would be made our subject. It's all in the biblical story of the Creation. Now we have to deal with the consequences.

It seems that Western culture lacks the foresight (an ability of the Liver) and the power (an ability primarily of the Gall Bladder, Stomach, and Spleen, but also of the Kidney as our will to survive) to change the course of environmental destruction quickly.

What to do? It seems that we have to rely on ourselves. But most of us do not have the power to bring a dead river back to life. Most of us do not have the power to force industries to be more conscious of nature. Most of us are not able to get rid of our poisonous cars, trucks, and airplanes overnight. Our economy has become so complex, and the individual branches so dependant on each other, that any sudden change threatens our survival. But our survival instincts were shaped in a different environment, in a different age. What helped us then can destroy us tomorrow. Our basic security patterns are not clever enough. It seems that we have to gather all of our intelligence to come to new—or very old—solutions fast.

How can we reverse our separation from nature? On the one hand, we can put all of our energy into seeing that changes occur. We can change ourselves and our lives so that we use fewer consumer goods and do without vicarious thrills. We can buy only one car, television set, and video recorder per family; we can drive less often, eat less meat, and take fewer pharmaceutical products. We can choose new goals that satisfy our body, mind, and soul in equal measure—goals that are not as destructive to the environment. We can learn to give each other a massage instead of driving to the disco 40 miles away on Saturday night. We can ride a bicycle to do errands instead of doing a workout on the home-fitness equipment or driving the car three blocks to the gym. We have already heard many of these suggestions.

On the other hand, it seems that we have to change a bit more than a few of our deeds and actions. It seems that we also have to undergo an inner process to become reconciled with nature in ourselves. It seems that we have to make our peace with nature. Earth is the Mother, not an enemy. It seems that we have to become reconciled with our emotions, with our fantasies and dreams, with our spiritual being. If we are not in tune with nature in ourselves, how can we act in the outside world to save the planet? As long as we fight the animal part of ourselves, how can we sincerely develop the sympathy necessary to save all the endangered species? As long as we forget about the plant part of ourselves—that quiescent and meditative part—how can we develop the love necessary to fight for all the endangered species?

It seems that, as we are all parts of the "iceberg," we need to start trusting nature again, we need to become again familiar with the elements. And it seems that we have to start with ourselves, spending more time fulfilling the basic needs of our body and soul in order to make possible a return to the essence of life.

Appendix

CLASSIFICATION BY THE FIVE ELEMENTS

	Wood	Fire	Earth	Metal	Water
Yin/Yang	young Yang	old Yang	neutral	young Yin	old Yin
Movement	expansion	vertically upward	horizontal here and there	concentration	vertically downward
Direction	east	south	middle	west	north
Season	spring	summer	late summer	fall	winter
Weather	windy	hot	humid	dry ·	cold
Energetic Character	tepid, mild, warm	steaming hot	neutralizing	cooling	bitter cold and frozen
Time of day	morning	midday	afternoon	evening	night
Life Cycle	birth and growth	blossoming	ripening and change	late ripening and decline	stagnation and down-fall
Use of the energy to:	sprout	blossom	ripen	harvest	store
Astrological Yang-Animal	tiger	horse	dog/sheep	rooster	bear
Astrological Yin-Animal	rabbit	snake	ox/dragon	ape	rat
Yang-Numbers	3	7	5	9	1

continues

133

	Wood	Fire	Earth	Metal	Water
Yin-Numbers	8	2	10	4	6
The Five *Zang*	liver	heart	spleen/ pancreas	lungs	kidneys
The Five *Fu*	gall bladder	small intestine	stomach	large intestine	bladder
Tissue	muscles and tendons	blood vessels	connecting tissue	skin	bones and bone marrow
Sensory Organs	eyes	tongue	mouth	nose	ears
The Five Senses	seeing	speaking	touching	tasting and smelling	hearing
Bodily Fluid	tears	perspiration	saliva and lymph	mucus	urine
Expression of Energy	nails	complexion	lips	body hair	hair (head)
Color	green	red	yellow and brown	white	blue and black
Complexion When Ill	light green, olive	mixture of red and white	yellowish	pale	dirty gray, dark brown
Smell When Ill	sour, rancid	burned, singed	unpleasantly sweet	smokey, spoiled, fishy	rotten, decayed
Behavior When Stressed	control	sadness and worry	stubborn, rigid, belching	denial; cough	shaking
Emotion	anger and rage	joy	compassion and caring	grief	fear
Tone of Voice	loud shouting	laughing, giggling	melodic singing	whining	groaning, deep voice
Predominant Temperament	choleric	sanguine, joyful	phlegmatic, compulsive	melancholic, discouraged	fearful, paranoid

continues

	Wood	Fire	Earth	Metal	Water
Elemental Spirit	*Hun:* soul, vision, inspiration	*Shen:* consciousness, love	*Yi:* intellect, practical intelligence	*Po:* instinct	*Zhen:* will to live, libido
Functions of the Elemental Spirit	plans and decisions, organization	integration, refinement, leadership	reflection, memory	concentration, analytical thinking	awe, meditation
Form of Energy	spiritual	psychological	physical	vital	ancestral
Influence of the Element on:	development of the physical	energy flow through the meridians	development of body form and consistency	rhythm of contraction and expansion	imagination, fantasy
Form of Therapy to Strengthen the Elements	sports, karate, *Tai Ji,* etc.	psychotherapy, moxibustion, acupuncture	diet and massage	breath therapy Rebirthing, Bach Flower Remedies	Hypnotherapy, Yoga, meditation
Dream	forest, trees	fire, laughter	singing, music	flying	drowning
Analysis	fighting	crowds	eating, drinking,	white objects	ocean, ships
(Examples)	shooting		heaviness	sky	
Flavor	sour	bitter	sweet	spicy	salty
Grain	wheat, rye	corn	millet	rice, oats	beans
Fruits	plums, berries	apricots	dates	peaches	grapes
Preparation	steam	eat raw	stew, roast	bake	grill
Tonifying	licorice	ginseng	orange peel	cayenne	marshmallow
Sedating	sage	caraway	basil	ginger, garlic	parsley

Bibliography

Academy of Traditional Chinese Medicine, *An Outline of Chinese Acupuncture*, Foreign Language Press, Beijing, China, 1975

Capra, Fritjof, *The Turning Point*, Bantam Books, New York, 1984

Connelly, Dianne, *Traditional Acupuncture*, Traditional Acupuncture Institute, Columbia, Maryland, 1994

Eckert, Achim, *Das Tao der Medizin* (*The Tao of Medicine*), Haug Verlag, Heidelberg, Germany, 1996

Gach, Michael, *Acu-Yoga*, Japan Publications, New York, 1981

Huang Ti Nei Ching Su Wen *The Yellow Emperor's Classic of Internal Medicine* (translated by Ilza Veith), University of California Press, Berkeley, California, 1972

Illich, Ivan, *Medical Nemesis: The Expropriation of Health*, Pantheon Books, New York, 1982

Jayasuriya, Anton, *Anatomy of Acupuncture*, Acupuncture Foundation of Sri Lanka, Colombo, 1979

Jayasuriya, Anton, *Clinical Acupuncture*, Acupuncture Foundation of Sri Lanka, Colombo, 1980

Lao-tse, *Tao Te King* (translated by Gia-Fu Feng and Jane English), Hugendubel, Munich, Germany, 1986

Lawson-Wood D. and J., *The Five Elements of Acupuncture and Chinese Massage*, Health Science Press, Rustington, England, 1965

Muramotu N., *Healing Ourselves*, Avon Books, New York, 1973

Needham, Joseph, *Science in Traditional China*, Harvard University Press, Cambridge, Massachussetts, 1982

Woollerton H. and McLean C., *Acupuncture Energy in Health and Disease*, Weatherby Woolnought, Wellingborough, England, 1979

Worsley, J. R., *Acupuncture: Is it for you?*, Element Books, Rockport, Massachusetts, 1991

Zukav, Gary, *The Dancing Wu Li Masters*, Morrow Quill Paperback Edition, New York, 1979

Index

Shiatsu for Beginners

Nigel Dawes
$16.95

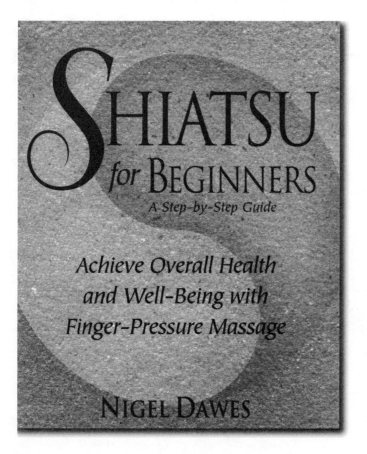

Shiatsu for Beginners intro-
duces American readers to
the ancient Japanese system
of pressure massage.
Shiatsu is an ancient,
gentle healing art of
applying pressure to the
body's energy channels
with fingers, thumbs,
hands, elbows, or knees.
This safe, holistic practice
balances the body's energy
and promotes good health.
Easy to learn and
rewarding to share, shiatsu
is a natural path to
relaxation and vitality.

To Order Books

Please send me the following items:

Quantity	Title	Unit Price	Total
_____	_____	$ _____	$ _____
_____	_____	$ _____	$ _____
_____	_____	$ _____	$ _____
_____	_____	$ _____	$ _____
_____	_____	$ _____	$ _____

Subtotal $ _____

Deduct 10% when ordering 3-5 books $ _____

7.25% Sales Tax (CA only) $ _____

8.25% Sales Tax (TN only) $ _____

5.0% Sales Tax (MD and IN only) $ _____

Shipping and Handling* $ _____

Total Order $ _____

Shipping and Handling depend on Subtotal.

Subtotal	Shipping/Handling
$0.00–$14.99	$3.00
$15.00–$29.99	$4.00
$30.00–$49.99	$6.00
$50.00–$99.99	$10.00
$100.00–$199.99	$13.50
$200.00+	Call for Quote

Foreign and all Priority Request orders:
Call Order Entry department
for price quote at 916/632-4400

This chart represents the total retail price of books only
(before applicable discounts are taken).

By Telephone: With MC or Visa, call 800-632-8676, 916-632-4400. Mon-Fri, 8:30-4:30.
WWW {http://www.primapublishing.com}

Orders Placed Via Internet E-mail {sales@primapub.com}
By Mail: Just fill out the information below and send with your remittance to:

**Prima Publishing
P.O. Box 1260BK
Rocklin, CA 95677**

My name is _____

I live at _____

City_____ State_____ Zip _____

MC/Visa#_____ Exp._____

Check/Money Order enclosed for $ _____Payable to Prima Publishing

Daytime Telephone _____

Signature _____